Sketches of Broken Minds

Sketches of Broken Minds

Nia Davies Williams

The manufacturer's authorised representative in the EU for product safety is Authorised Rep
Compliance Ltd, 71 Lower Baggot Street, Dublin D02 P593 Ireland
(www.arccompliance.com)

Troubador Publishing Ltd
Unit E2 Airfield Business Park,
Harrison Road, Market Harborough,
Leicestershire. LE16 7UL
Tel: 0116 2792299
Email: books@troubador.co.uk
Web: www.troubador.co.uk

ISBN 978 1836282 174

British Library Cataloguing in Publication Data.
A catalogue record for this book is available from the British Library.

Printed and bound in Great Britain by 4edge Limited
Typeset in 11pt Minion Pro by Troubador Publishing Ltd, Leicester, UK

*Dedicated to all the people living with dementia with
whom I have shared the joy that music can bring*

Contents

Preface

'When words fail, music speaks'.
(Hans Christian Anderson)

This book has been written as a record of my experiences, as a musician, of working with people who have succumbed to the debilitating effects of dementia at various stages of the disease. Many of these individuals are people with whom I have worked with for many months, or in some cases, several years. This is not an academic book or a book that explores the scientific side of dementia. Rather, it is a book that is based on one musician's observational experiences of the disease and how music can combat some of its problems in often strange and mysterious ways. The book also includes chapters on day-to-day observations of the lives of people living with dementia.

When I started keeping a diary of my experiences a few years ago, two scientists visited the dementia care centre where I mainly worked to observe one of my music sessions. They were conducting some research for a radio programme they were presenting on the development of the brain and the many subsequent causes of its deterioration. During a discussion at the end of the session, I told them that I felt the need to research my findings and wished I had the kind of scientific background in neuroscience and psychology that would have enabled me to delve into the scientific side of my findings. One of the scientists turned round to me and said, 'You should just carry on doing what you are doing here. It's important that you document your observations and let people see what you are doing. Let the scientists take care of the science behind it!'

This was the kind of confirmation I needed to continue with my goal of writing a book on the first-hand experiences of a musician working in this area. I therefore see this book as a record of how people with dementia respond to music, and other art forms, in very different and often very revealing ways. I shall indeed leave the science to the scientists.

However, in order to understand the relationship between dementia and music, and to put my book in context, I start with a short introduction which attempts to chart the relationship between scientific research, music and dementia. Explanations will be given on certain behaviours that lie behind the various forms of dementia that relate to certain residents whose conditions I have observed over time. The introduction is designed to help support and explain some findings and observations made later on in this book.

Another point worth noting here is the *kind* of research used in this field. When I was studying for my masters' degree some years ago, I had to write a thesis on the research that I had completed during my work as a coordinator and co-leader of one of the Alzheimer's Society's *Singing for the Brain* sessions. I had used a mixed approach of qualitative and quantitative research.[1] However, a substantial part of recording the actual sessions involved forms of *narrative* research; in other words, observing and writing out what actually took place.[2] When I showed some of my narrative research to one of my supervisors, she became critical of my work. She said that it was *too* narrative and not 'scientific' enough. I had to make the argument that – in this context – the narrative approach was indeed a useful and entirely acceptable form of research.

One need look no further than the writings of the eminent neurologist Oliver Sacks (1933–2015), who on several occasions lamented the fact that narrative research had gradually disappeared from the pages of scholarly texts during the twentieth century. Sacks argued that while the narrative approach had been largely overtaken by scientific discourse, there was still so much that could be learnt from the former. In fact, during the eighteenth and nineteenth centuries, narrative research was *de rigueur*. Scientists would often record and document their observations in great detail. The research was

1   Qualitative Research is exploratory, providing a detailed description of the research topic. Quantitative Research is more statistical and deals with facts and figures that explain what is observed.

2   Narrative research focuses on the real-life experiences of individuals. It tries to gather an understanding of the subject, and present its findings, through a narrative account of what happened.

interesting to read and future scientists would learn from these observations.

This book is therefore written as a narrative account of the relationship between music and people who have dementia. The evidence provided is therefore mainly anecdotal: a narrative of my work and findings in this area. In his book *In Pursuit of Memory: The Fight Against Alzheimer's,* Joseph Jebelli points out that observation through anecdotal evidence has an important part to play in such research, and should not be overlooked:

> *In the rigorous, dispassionate realm of academia, anecdotal evidence is often given short shrift. It suffers mainly from having no experimental 'control' – no objective means of comparison, that is – to minimise variables and increase scientific objectivity. We depend on controls to infer whether two things are causally linked. But … anecdotes sometimes have another power. They can lead to new hypotheses. They can take what seems absurd and use it to arouse creativity.*[3]

Therefore, if anecdotal evidence or narrative research is recognised as being worthwhile in a field such as dementia studies, then clearly more of it is needed. To carers looking after loved ones or people working in this sector in various roles, my message to them is this: if you have a few minutes to spare after a hard days' or nights'

---

3   Joseph Jebelli, *In Pursuit of Memory: The Fight Against Alzheimer's* (John Murray, 2017), p. 162.

work, document your experiences and findings – for you will never know what may come of those findings in the future.

The utmost respect has been afforded to the privacy of the residents and families who appear in this book. Original names of residents and families have been replaced with pseudonyms. No direct background details have been disclosed that would expose residents or their families unless approved by the next of kin. Written consent relating to materials and photographs published in this book has been given by the next of kin.

Introduction

The most appropriate way to describe people who have dementia is as exactly that: people who have dementia or people living with dementia. The abbreviation PWD – people with dementia – will be used throughout this book. While dementia is without doubt a terrible and debilitating disease and one that still remains at present largely incurable, the term 'sufferer' should almost certainly be avoided when talking about PWD. For those people who receive medical care, as is the case with those who live in nursing rather than residential homes, we should always refer to them as 'patients'.

To my mind, a rather annoying term that has crept into recent discourse on PWD, especially in the private care sector, is 'client'. In pseudo-economic speak, this is presumably meant to express a kind of 'business' arrangement that exists between the patient/client and the care home, centre or sector that looks after the person. Clearly, PWD are not *clients* of dementia, and I will refrain from using this term. To me, PWD are not clients – there is no transaction between the care home or nursing home that the residents are themselves aware of. They are in the care home to be cared for. Oliver Sacks also disagreed with the use of the word 'clients' in this context, stating: '"clients" (an odious word … supposedly less degrading than "patients")'.[4]

As stated in the Preface, this book is not intended as a scientific study of music and dementia. For example, patients were not wired up and functional MRI scans conducted while music was played in the background with the results subsequently being fed into a computer database for analysis and processing. If it isn't already taking place, then certainly there's room for this kind of research in the future. But not here. However, while taking an avowedly non-scientific approach, it is nevertheless necessary for readers to familiarise themselves with some of the most common terms associated with dementia to help understand and explain the patterns of behaviour and responses of some of the residents discussed in this book.[5]

Dementia is the term given to describe a multitude of diseases that affects the brain. The most common forms of dementia, affecting most of the residents mentioned in this book, are provided in the following list:

---

4   Oliver Sacks, *The Man Who Mistook his Wife for a Hat* (Picador Classics, 1985), p. 174.
5   The exact form of dementia is not given to all of whom are mentioned in this book. In the case of some residents, it is not known exactly what kind of dementia that person may actually have.

Alzheimer's. The most common form of dementia. A slightly higher percentage of women suffer from this form of dementia. The main symptoms are difficulty remembering names and recent events, along with apathy and depression. As the disease progresses, symptoms such as impaired judgment, disorientation, confusion and behavioural changes appear. Further into the development, the individual will have difficulty speaking, swallowing and walking.

Early onset Alzheimer's. Anyone with dementia, including Alzheimer's, before the age of 65 falls into this category. In some cases, it can include people who are in their early 50s or even in their 40s. Unless caused by external factors such as lifestyle (alcoholism or drug abuse, for example), or suffering a serious accident, early onset dementia can be hereditary. There is some evidence that the progression of dementia is more rapid in the cases of early onset.

Vascular dementia. This is the second commonest form of dementia, affecting more men than women. This type of dementia occurs from blood vessel blockage or damage leading to strokes or bleeding in the brain. Symptoms here include impaired judgment or lack of ability to plan the necessary steps required to complete a task.

Dementia with Lewy bodies. As is the case with people with Alzheimer's, those who have dementia with Lewy bodies often suffer from memory loss and thinking problems, but they may also experience symptoms such as sleep disturbances, well-formed visual hallucinations, slowness, gait imbalance or other physical movement features associated with Parkinson's disease.

Frontotemporal dementia. Typical symptoms here include changes in personality and behaviour and difficulty with language, which is sometimes referred to as *aphasia*.

Mixed dementia. Many more people have been diagnosed with *mixed dementia* in recent years, suggesting that the condition is more common than previously thought. Symptoms are a simultaneous combination of other forms of dementia, for example, Alzheimer's and Vascular dementia.

Alcohol-related brain damage such as Korsakoff (or Wernicke-Korsakoff) Syndrome. A chronic memory disorder most often caused by alcohol misuse and subsequent lack of thiamine. It affects short-term memory but also produces gaps in long-term memory. It can also cause unsteadiness and problems processing new information.

In order to properly comprehend the purpose and intended value of this book, it is important that the reader remains receptive and open to the notion that music and the other arts can be beneficial to patients living with dementia. Only by accepting the positive and powerful hold that music in particular exerts on PWD can we start to ascertain and appreciate its efficacious effect through the many music sessions that I have held from week to week for many years. With this in mind, a brief review of some of the key research questions in relation to music and dementia is set out for those who'd like to know more about the relationship between music and dementia.

Experts such as music therapists David Aldridge, Gudrun Aldridge and the neurologist Oliver Sacks have claimed for many years that those areas of the brain that deal with music are one of the last parts to be affected by a disease such as Alzheimer's. These are the areas that first develop in childhood because the roots of language are musical. Aldridge reports as follows:

> *Although language deterioration is a feature of cognitive deficit, musical abilities appear to be preserved. This may be because the fundamentals of language itself are musical and are prior to semantic and lexical functions in language development.*[6]

While language processing takes place mainly in one hemisphere of the brain (the left side), music involves an understanding between both sides of the cerebral hemisphere. Sacks's research suggests that the areas of the brain that deal with music are spared to a large degree with the onset of dementia and are therefore different to those parts that deal only with language processing and verbal communication. Music therapist Robin Rio has also acknowledged that music utilizes many different areas of the brain:

---

6   David Aldridge, 'Two Epistemologies: Music Therapy and Medicine in the Treatment of Dementia', *The Arts in Psychotherapy*, Vol. 19 (1992), p. 247.

The incredible thing about music is that, perhaps because of its holistic nature, requiring many areas of the brain and body to work simultaneously, it can sometimes bypass some of the debilitating condition and allow the healthier parts of the brain to take over.[7]

As a result, an individual's musical capabilities are largely preserved, even though memory and the ability to use language may deteriorate. And even when the ability to identify a song disappears, the ability to emotionally respond to it will continue.

In his book *And Still the Music Plays*, Graham Stokes, an internationally recognised authority on dementia care practice and policy, claims that our earliest experiences form a strong part of our mental makeup. Experiences that happened so early on in our lives that we cannot even recollect them – such as a mother singing a lullaby to her infant child – remain embedded in our memories. In Stokes's words:

What happens prior to our earliest accessible memories is laid down as personal truth. It is just what we know about ourselves, the way we are. The question is can we forget that which is not remembered? Can we lose that which has not been laid down as an accessible memory trace? The answer is, in all likelihood, no.[8]

---

7   Robin Rio, *Connecting Through Music with People with Dementia: A Guide for Caregivers* (Jessica Kingsley Publishers, 2009), p. 94.
8   Graham Stokes, *And Still the Music Plays: Stories of People with Dementia* (Hawker Publications, 2009), p. 106.

In other words, Stokes states that we do not make a conscious effort to learn and remember the songs and music we hear when we are just a few weeks or months old; rather, they became part of our very makeup: gold nuggets of sensory experience that lie buried in the memory bank from virtually one's first breath of life.

The above research asserts that one's musical abilities appear to be preserved and that this has a unique effect on PWD. Music can therefore be used as an alternate way for PWD to communicate – to be soothed or stimulated in addition to reigniting cognitive aspects such as memory. Rio explains that the process of transferring information from short term into long term memory is affected by a disease that causes dementia (such as Alzheimer's) to such an extent that the ability to learn something new becomes very limited. Nevertheless, Rio notes that some issues can be helpful here:

> *Things that may improve this absorption of short-term events into the long-term memory are: associations with the other known things; an emotional reaction or enhanced mood; repetition; organisation and categorisation of information; the information having meaning; and information being provided with humour. This explains a lot of why music can be easier to remember than some other things.*[9]

Elsewhere, Hays and Minichiello's research looks at the significance of music in the lives of the elderly, including

---

9   Robin Rio, *Connecting Through Music with People with Dementia: A Guide for Caregivers* (Jessica Kingsley Publishers, 2009), pp. 91–92.

PWD. Their conclusions highlight the importance of music for the individual's self-respect, his or her wellbeing, their ability to connect with others, and a means of avoiding feelings of loneliness:

Music is an important part of the lives of people because it is through music that they can come to know and reflect upon their own personhood.[10]

Most people have acquired at one time or another an emotional attachment and reaction to certain types of music. These are forever linked together. Just think of the popular BBC4 radio program *Desert Island Discs* to appreciate how a song or a musical composition is often linked to an important moment or experience in a person's life.

With this in mind, part of my work involves spending time talking to colleagues and carers, families and friends, carrying out research into the musical preferences of PWD and the likely connotations that hearing or singing along with those musical preferences may invoke in the residents themselves. By discovering what kinds of music each individual enjoys – which songs they listened to when they were children, during the first flush of youth, or when they got married and had children – this information will enable the musician working in a care home to elicit the most effective response and reactions to music sessions.

---

10   T. Hays and V. Minichiello, 'The meaning of music in the lives of older people: a qualitative study', *Psychology of Music*, 33 (2005), p. 440.

The PWD's memory of these periods in their lives – the rites of passage that often comprise childhood, youth, marriage and the start of family life – are often clearer when happy memories are made, as it can quite often be accompanied by a period in a person's life of stability, good health and general wellbeing. I recently saw an advertisement for some kind of health drink that claimed benefits for a healthy brain: 'Insure your memories', it said. If only this were possible!

One final point, obvious but nevertheless worth mentioning, is that I work with people who – most often than not – I have not known as the person they were before the onset of dementia. I have never known the diligent and capable nurse or the caring family doctor behind the dementia, the strict but respected head teacher, the highly regarded councillor or the loving housewife. But I always make every effort to try to find that person. And sometimes, often in the course of conducting a music session, glimpses of that person will shine through.

Suddenly the character of the original person will appear from behind the mask of memory loss. It saddens me that some carers in a care home often do not have the time to sit and talk with residents, taking proper time to find the person behind the dementia. I know this can be difficult, especially for those in the later stages of dementia, but music can certainly play a part in bringing out the person who still exists behind the condition. While those memories may be broken and fragmentary, they are still accessible, and music is often the only key that is capable of unlocking them.

As mentioned earlier, certain songs can help specific PWD reminisce, and often, as a result, the conversation becomes clearer and the resident more coherent and lucid. An avenue of communication is often opened and established through music. This allows the resident or visiting musician to enter the world of the person sitting there and begin the often very rewarding and valuable process of getting to know the person behind the dementia.

1. Prologue: Hands on Music

The people who form the subjects of this book are either residential care or nursing care residents. Those who are in residential care are usually people with early- to mid-stage dementia. Most can use the bathroom independently or with a little help. They can eat their meals mostly unaided and can get themselves dressed with guidance or assistance.

Nursing care residents usually have mid- to late-stage dementia and/or growing physical needs. A hoist may be required to lift them to and from a bed or chair; they may need the use of a wheelchair for mobility or require a walking aid such as a frame. Nursing care residents are often dependent on help with personal care and during mealtimes. A nurse will be available twenty-four hours of every single day to administer medication.

Some residents are moved from residential care to nursing care as the symptoms of their dementia develops. One such resident was Mavis. I came across Mavis around 10 years ago when she was moved from residential care to nursing care, not because her dementia was progressing but because of physical deterioration – her worsening arthritis was making movement particularly painful. Mavis could walk with the aid of a frame when she arrived at the care home, but after a few months this would continually get harder and more painful for her until she could only move with the aid of a hoist and wheelchair.

Some residents cope better than others with the use of a hoist. However, for Mavis, it was very upsetting for her no matter how reassuring the carers were, and she could be heard down the hallway, calling out in distress. This was made slightly more bearable for her if she was told that she would then be going to a music session, as Mavis enjoyed music and singing very much. She would attend most group sessions, knowing and enjoying most of the Welsh songs we would sing, from folk songs such as '*Yr Eneth Gaeth ei Gwrthod*' (The Rejected Maiden) and '*Mae Nghariad i'n Fenws*' (My Love is a Venus) to hymns such as '*Calon Lân*' (Pure Heart) and '*Pererin Wyf*' (Amazing Grace).

During these singing sessions, Mavis would sit in a chair with her arms crossed, tucking her hands into the sleeves of her cardigan, which gave her some comfort. As the music started Mavis would inevitably join in the singing, releasing her hands from the sleeves of her cardigan and start rubbing them together, not so much to the rhythm of the music but to the actual melody. For example, during a rendition of Jean Sibelius' hymn 'Finlandia'[11] instead of beating time to the music she would turn her hands over and over in keeping with the melody. Not only did Mavis know every word, but she also knew every note of the melody and its rhythm too.

Many PWD will revert to the language of their childhood as the disease progresses, so a PWD born into a Welsh-speaking family but married to an English partner and having lived for most of his/her life in England with English-speaking children will quite possibly start speaking in Welsh again.

However, this is not always the case. Mavis was born and raised into a Welsh family, married a Welsh husband and raised her two sons through the medium of Welsh. She lived all her life in a predominantly Welsh-speaking rural area in North Wales. Her parents kept a small grocery shop and Mavis had to help during the war by driving the delivery van full of groceries. Nearly all her parents' customers would have spoken Welsh, so why did Mavis now speak mainly in English even though most of the carers spoke to her in Welsh? Could it be that she sensed that she was not 'at home' – that the people around her were strangers to her and that she always spoke to strangers in English?

Or could it be something else perhaps? Mavis was born in the early 1920s, and she would have attended a school where the educational system of the time was almost

---

11   Hymn version, set to Welsh words by the poet and playwright Saunders Lewis.

entirely conducted through the English language. Children were not allowed to speak Welsh in the classroom and were even discouraged from speaking the language in the playground. By reverting to the language of her childhood, was this not therefore, for Mavis, English? Perhaps, in her mind she imagined that the nursing home was a Welsh school from the 1920s. We can never know the reasoning for sure, only continue to make the effort to understand.

2. Living Well with Dementia?

In February 2009, a national dementia strategy was published by the British government entitled 'Living Well with Dementia'. Its main aim was to set out a 'vision for transforming dementia services with the aim of achieving better awareness of dementia, early diagnosis and high quality treatment at whatever stage of the illness and in whatever setting.'[12] The strategy signalled a change in emphasis and attitude, not only from dementia services but also within the NHS, where the focus shifted onto the individuals themselves and on the importance of 'Living Well with Dementia' through maintaining and continuing a social life, keeping active, occupied and combating sleep problems.

For PWD, achieving the goal of living well with dementia may be 'easier' to do so from the familiar surroundings of one's own home and with the care and support of a loved one. But sometimes this is not always possible. It becomes

---

12   <https://www.gov.uk/government/news/living-well-with-dementia-a-national-dementia-strategy> accessed 29 July 2018.

very hard for a loved one to care for a PWD because of his or her declining mental as well as physical health. The carer may herself or himself be elderly, and themselves not in the best of health, and after much agonising and deliberation they will come to the inevitable conclusion that there are no viable options other than to turn to a care home or nursing home for support. One such example was Marjorie and her husband.

*****

Marjorie's husband, who was himself in his nineties, would drive a fair distance every morning to the care home where she resided. He would do this mainly to make sure that Marjorie attended the music sessions. He would arrive punctually at the home, make his way to the lounge, then escort his wife to the music room by himself. They would walk hand in hand, both of them slowly making their way over, with words of encouragement from him all the way until Marjorie was seated comfortably in her favourite spot by the large window overlooking the gardens.

I was quite touched by this little routine of care that took so much effort on his behalf. I also found it endearing that every time he turned to leave after kissing Marjorie goodbye, she would always come out with a comment such as, 'Pull your jumper down at the back, dear', or 'Fasten up your cardigan, dear'. And he would always respond sincerely with 'Yes, dear. Does that look alright now?' There was never even a sigh of annoyance, just quiet compliance and acceptance.

As my role as musician usually involves working with people of a certain age, I sometimes get a glimpse of how a special relationship between husband and wife can last for such a long time. Most importantly, their respect for each other is never lost. Love for the complete person is also vitally important, of course. And patience, as we know, is a virtue. I guess one either learns to live with certain things, or one doesn't. Certainly, love and respect on behalf of both husband and wife will go a very long way into securing a long and happy relationship.

I noticed that Marjorie had not been attending many music sessions over a period of a few weeks, and when I went in search of her, I found her sitting in the corner of the lounge having a snooze after finishing her breakfast. It transpired that the carers had not seen her husband for several days. Apparently, he had been taken ill and had been spending time in hospital. I immediately got on the phone and called him.

The voice on the other side of the phone sounded frail and weak. It was clear that he had not been well for some time. But he said he was getting a little stronger day-by-day. 'I'm not quite strong enough to drive over just yet, but as soon as I can, I'll come and visit Marjorie.'

I promised her husband that we would take good care of Marjorie, ensuring that she continued to attend as many music sessions as possible. This seemed to reassure him, as he always felt very strongly that Marjorie benefitted a lot from attending the sessions and was desperate for her to be involved. 'You see, Marjorie loves music and singing. I've noticed that she remembers the words to many songs. It's important that she doesn't lose that ability.'

During the months that followed, there were many times when Marjorie's husband became too unwell to visit his wife. For Marjorie, it was her mental faculties that had deserted her. For Marjorie's husband, it was his body that was gradually deteriorating. But as soon as he was strong enough, he would came back to her. And their little routine would start over again, both of them a little frailer each time …

*****

I have seen some cases of people who appear to be 'living well with dementia' in care homes and nursing homes. Certainly keeping active and occupied and having some form of social life, even if it's just coming together for a small 'in-house' concert with other residents, can contribute towards living well with dementia. Some residents embrace the activities that go on in care and nursing homes. These residents will engage well with the carers and nurses overall, and as a result, will often become well-loved by members of staff, from the cleaners and caterers to the carers and nurses and even amongst administrative staff. They will seem content – smiling, singing and eating well.

In one particularly large care home there lived a man called Bobby. Everybody seemed to know Bobby, from all the staff to most of the care home's regular visitors. Bobby had mid- to late-stage Alzheimer's and would often be seen shuffling along the hallways, smiling, often humming a tune to himself. He would eat well, enjoying the attention given to him by carers and visitors, and would be happy to attend music sessions and concerts. Like many others with dementia, he seemed to have managed to completely let go of any worries. Living as they do for – and in – the moment, some PWD do not seem to be worried about anything. They don't fret or seem anxious or become upset.

Another gentleman, called Mathew,[13] had early- to mid-stage dementia. He was aware that he had dementia. He would often comment, while pointing to his head: 'I have this dementia you know. That's why I'm here. It can be a blooming nuisance. You're going to have to remind me when you have your music sessions … I don't want to miss one!' Mathew used to be a trumpet player and was very keen on the music sessions. His knowledge of music, especially trumpet players, was impressive. Even though Mathew seemed to be aware of his condition, he seemed to have settled well in the nursing home. He connected well with the carers and enjoyed his meals. He would go for short walks and attend any sessions that involved music.

However, unfortunately many more PWD do nothing but worry and fret during the whole of their waking hours. They cling onto their worries like a lead raft that seems to plunge them further and deeper into the dark abyss, as the next chapter will highlight.

---

13   There is more about Mathew later, in the chapter entitled 'The Jazz Man and the Trumpet Man'.

3. On a Loop

Unfortunately, I see many more examples of people 'not living well with dementia' than the opposite case. They can be heard calling out repeatedly for their mothers or daughters, fathers or sons, terrified. Crying, shaking, lost – they can be seen wondering endlessly around the corridors of the care home. One lady would walk around, ceaselessly crying out: 'I'm dying! Dying to go home! I'm sick, I'm homesick!' Some become closed off from the outside world, retreating further and further into their own shell, consoling themselves repeatedly with words of comfort that one might use to console a child. Many PWD will reiterate the same phrases over and over. They may repeat a very short comment or a series of numbers, a line from a song or a few words from a poem. It can be a question asked over and over again, a statement or a command.

Robert turned up one day at the home looking very dapper, clothes well matched, shoes polished, shirt pressed and a perfectly knotted tie around his neck. Every hair was in place. The perfect image of a gentleman. But Robert soon became quite fretful, walking the hallways for hours every day. This pattern escalated over the course of many months, as his overall health deteriorated further. The clothes that were once so neat and tidy when he first arrived now hung loosely around his body. He was reduced to skin and bones. Despite the carers' attempts to coax and cajole him into eating his meals, he would hardly sit down for more than a few minutes before rising up again, a worried look upon his face, before taking yet another journey down the long corridors of the home.

Soon after this, Robert started to recite the words to the popular Welsh hymn 'Calon Lân' (Pure Heart) on a constant loop for days on end. The days then turned into weeks. Popular Welsh hymns were one of the very few things from which he still found a crumb of comfort and enjoyment. One afternoon when Robert was particularly fretful, continually reciting the words to the same hymn, I managed to coax him over to the music room where I started playing some of his favourite hymns on the piano. To begin with, he sat down beside me and sang along to the hymns, but still wore the same worried look on his face. Then, after a short while, he stood up and shuffled around the room for a little while before joining me again by the piano to sing a little more. I was glad to see and hear him singing something different to the usual repetitive phrases and remark on how well he knew the words to all these hymns.

However, following our little one-to-one session, Robert immediately went back to reciting the words to 'Calon

Lân', even though I had deliberately avoided singing that particular hymn with him, hoping against hope that I could somehow bring him out of the constant loop that seemed to punish and comfort him at the same time. Robert continued in this way for weeks and months, grinding himself down, until his voice eventually became weak and hoarse, slowing right down and almost to a halt – as if a long-life battery in his body was finally running out of charge.

What quality of life did this man have? Some may consider this a controversial suggestion, but surely giving Robert something to help him sleep away some of those dreadful hours would have been better than living in a constant fretful state and with a restless mind that refused to give his mind and body the rest it so sorely needed.

Like Robert, many residents will wander around the care home. It is a symptom of their dementia. It can be quite difficult to involve such residents in music as they are upwardly mobile most of the day. To try and reach them, I'll sometimes play music on the piano with the music room door propped open. With residents who constantly wander aimlessly around the corridors and hallways of their care home, they are sometimes drawn to the music and will walk into the music room for a while before they resume their roaming around. After a while, these familiar faces will come round again, wandering back into the music room. They will sometimes walk in on a group session, stay a short while, before wandering off again. This is the closest I can get to a music session with some

PWD. I'll occasionally play my Celtic harp in the hallways to the same effect.

*****

'91264!' called out Jenny when she often became distressed, reciting the phone number over and over. She thought she was calling for her parents. 'Mummy! Daddy! Where Are You?' The phone number had stuck forever in her fragmented memory. These fragments would often become stuck in the minds of people like Jenny like a scratched vinyl record stuck in a groove and unable to move forward. It's possible to distract a resident briefly with a song, a tune, or perhaps a little chat. But they will always revert: revert to their own cruel mantra, for which the only escape, ironically, is through further erosion and final deterioration that accompanies dementia's ominous march onwards.

Another female resident who would walk around the care home all day was Eleanor. She constantly repeated the words, 'I don't like it! I don't want it Mr Brown!' When someone would ask her 'Who is Mr Brown?', she would reflect the question back at the person by saying, 'Who is Mr Brown?' before resuming her set phrase over and over again. When you smiled at Eleanor, she'd smile back. Maybe she was simply emulating your smile, perhaps in the same way that she copied people's questions. In a strange way Eleanor's actions suggested that she was reverting to a child-like sensibility, imitating – like children often do – in order to learn. But the sad fact was that Eleanor was heading towards the end of her life. She was not at the beginning.

Maybe music could help. I decided to play out a musical game with Eleanor. When I sang a single note and held it, Eleanor would join in and copy me by singing the same note. I then tried another note – a little higher this time – and again, Eleanor sang the higher note with me, perfectly in tune. I tried various notes of various pitches and she'd 'tune into' each and every one of them.

It was uncanny how she managed to do this. One morning, I heard Eleanor singing to herself quite contently with simple 'La, la, la' words. But she couldn't go beyond the 'La- la's': she was caught in a 'La-la' loop. I walked along with her for a while before latching on to her 'La's' by gently singing the chorus from Raymond Wallace's 'Jolly Good Company': 'La-di-da-di-dah, La-di-da-di-dee. All good pals and jolly good company.' Eleanor joined in during the 'La-di-da-di-dah, La-di-da-di-dee'. We walked around the long hallways of the care home like this for quite a while with Eleanor joining in with the 'La-di-das', but when I eventually left her, she resorted back to her usual phrases.

One afternoon a few months later I was playing the little Celtic harp in a lounge at the same care home where Eleanor lived. Out of the corner of my eye, I'd noticed her passing the lounge many times on one of her never-ending walks, and as I sang 'My Bonnie Lies Over the Ocean', she came into the lounge and stood above me for a short while before starting to sing along to the chorus:

'Bring back, bring back,
Oh, bring back my Bonny to me, to me,
Bring back, bring back,
Oh, bring back my Bonny to me.'

Eleanor's husband would visit the home a couple of times every week, but he never managed to get any kind of conversation out of his wife. It was hard to ascertain if she even knew who he was. Eleanor would sometimes sit for a while and her husband would try talking to her but with hardly any reaction in return. Eventually, Eleanor's husband could be seen walking slowly back to his car, having again visited a person – his wife – who now regarded him as a complete stranger. There were no words of love or comfort for him. No words of recognition, even. The dementia had already taken his wife away.

*****

Amongst the many other examples of PWD 'stuck' in mind-numbing vocal patterns was a lady who would call out: 'NURSE! Come here and talk to me!' This happened even when the carer was in fact sitting right next to her, holding her hand, reassuring her. 'I'm here, right next to you'. A moment would pass, then again, she would call out: 'NURSE! Come here and talk to me!' The presence of a carer next to her did not deter the lady from calling out. The 'calling out' had now become an inextricable part of her character, an unwanted response mechanism and persistent habit that she simply couldn't shake off. Some nursing residents would often cry out, 'Help! Help!' Those individuals would be given reassurance and comfort, but then would call out again within seconds: 'Help! Help! HELP!'

Lost inside their own damaged minds, many of these residents had entered the twilight zone of their dementia – the final stages of a journey that offered little comfort, reassurance or hope. On the outside, many of them resembled a pitiful, shrunken husk of the person they used to be. But you must search for the person behind this cruel illness: through love, through patience, through talking, through music and even through humour. It's a wonderful moment when you manage to reconnect – when a shaft of recognition lights up inside the murky shadows of their memory. Even if it's just for a brief moment. Never let go, no matter how hard it may seem.

Although it's sometimes possible to distract PWDs from these continuous, repetitive utterances by getting them to join in with various sections from songs, they will inevitably resort back to their usual state. Their condition has become so deeply engrained in their minds that words and fragments of songs becomes a part of them.

Lavinia would sing the tune to the first two lines of 'Oh My Darling, Clementine' loudly, over and over. Her constant singing was so loud that I feared it would start to affect other residents in the lounge. They were battling their own confused and broken minds. I could see the look of desperation and fatigue etched upon their sallow faces. Some residents were frightful of Lavinia. Others shouted at her indignantly to be quiet. Those who could still walk unaided would shuffle down the hallway to get away from the constant noise.

Not that it was easy on the carers, either, in such trying circumstances, especially when the resident in question was subject to one-to-one care. Many would spend hours in the company of such residents, often with just short breaks. If I sang a different tune to Lavinia closely, near her ear, she would transfer from her repeated mantra of 'Oh My Darling, Clementine' to the song that I'd be singing, but would then immediately transfer back again to 'Clementine' once I'd finished singing.

With Mona, it was possible to have a little conversation to a degree, and she seemed quite content in the care home with her husband visiting regularly. He also felt that she seemed comfortable, content and as happy as one might expect a person to be under such circumstances. However, at one point Mona became ill. She contracted a chest infection and became bedridden for many weeks. There were times when it seemed that Mona would not recover, but she was still physically quite strong and recover she did.

But after getting better there was no longer any sort of conversation from Mona – no smiles and no acknowledgement of her husband's presence. She began to repeat herself in a constant loop. She would say, 'Try to tidy, tidy, tidy, tidy...' then stopping for a split second to take a sharp breath before continuing throughout her waking hours, '...Try to tidy, tidy, tidy, tidy...' By the end of the day, she'd tired herself out so much that her voice had become hoarse. There was desperation in her eyes and fatigue etched across her face. But she could not stop herself and on went the constant repetition. Sleep, at least, when it came, would bring with it some relief and a little peace until the next day, which would follow the same desperate pattern as the previous day.

Many residents will ask the same questions over and over again. At first, they are simply trying to make some sort of sense out of their confusion. In time, these questions will often turn into repetitive loops, ingraining themselves in the person's mind and becoming part of the very fabric of their spoken selves. Questions such as:

'Why am I here?' What is this place? Where is this place?'

'Do buses come by here? Where do they stop? When's the next one?'

'You see, I've got to get home now … my family will be wondering where I am …'

'Do you have a car? Do you drive to work? Can you give me a lift home?'

'I've got money, you know. Where's all my money? Who has all my money?'

PWD can become fixated by certain worries, and this will relay itself through these constant questions. Music can at least break the loop, for a short while.

4. Good Days, Bad Days

'And all my grief flows from the rift
Of unremembered skies and snows.'

('Clown in the Moon' by Dylan Thomas)

Of course, life with dementia is not always black and white. The people who seem to suffer the most will also have better days. They will smile when they feel the late summer sun on their faces or when they hear a favourite song being sung – just as those people who seem on the whole quite content and happy will have times when they become irritable, tearful or angry. This will often happen at the end of the day and is commonly known as the 'sundown syndrome'.[14]

Music can certainly help here. Around this time of the day, many of the residents seem to sense that not all is right in their world – a sudden moment of fearful clarity when they realise that they are in a care home because of their

---

14   Also sometimes referred to as 'sundowning', where PWD can become more agitated, aggressive or confused during early evening.

failing memory. At that point, all he or she will want to do is to be with her husband or his wife and go home to familiar surroundings. It can be very hard for a PWD to accept this situation. They can become distressed, upset, restless, vocal and angry.

Andrew was one such resident who would often become restless in the early evening. He had a lovely deep voice and would listen to music, joining in when we would sing Welsh hymns such as '*Calon Lân*' ('Pure Heart'). Andrew would usually be found in a jolly mood and in good spirits. But he would also become very tearful, and the sound of his own voice singing would – at times – make him very upset. Andrew's wife did not live nearby, but she would visit every day, spending hours by her husband's side chatting to him while maybe doing some knitting.

I discovered that Andrew enjoyed listening to jazz, so one morning – when Andrew was feeling particularly morose and melancholy – I brought out the iPad and went through a list of famous jazz musicians with him, from Miles Davis and Charlie Parker to Duke Ellington and Louis Armstrong, until I came across a particular piece that seemed to strike a chord with Andrew. His demeanour immediately changed at the sound of Armstrong's trumpet melody on Gershwin's famous tune 'Summertime', and he would relax back into his chair.

I took a photo of Andrew sitting back in his chair and showed it to his wife the next time she visited the home. There he was, listening with headphones to what was obviously a very enjoyable piece of music for him. The anxious face had been replaced by contentment – the dark shadow of doubt replaced by a knowing smile, along with the comfort and familiarity that sometimes only music can bring.

*****

For Evan, another resident in the same care home as Andrew, on particularly bad days it was the mornings that could be really challenging. Evan enjoyed a good old chat, especially if it was a conversation about his favourite football club, Everton – the team he had supported all his life. He also enjoyed and was particularly knowledgeable about poetry and music. Evan especially enjoyed popular Welsh music, but he also liked to listen to Elvis and the Rolling Stones. We'd sing our hearts out to some of Everton's football chants, much to Liverpool supporters' annoyance (their rival club) at the home!

However, on certain mornings Evan could be very vocal, shouting and quarrelling with fellow residents and being argumentative with the carers. There was no conversation – just accusations and berating. As the day wore on, Evan's temper would eventually subside, and I'd catch a glimpse of him as I'd be leaving the home at the end of the day, sitting, legs crossed, hands folded together on his lap, chatting happily to a family member, a visiting friend, or a carer. The storm raging inside him had subsided, and calm presided, at least momentarily; until the next time, which, with Evan, was unfortunately inevitable…

*****

Dorothea was both a very intelligent and highly determined lady. A retired school mistress, she would waste no time in correcting carers on grammar or how to lay out the table correctly. She was deaf in one ear and wore a hearing aid in the other, with which she would constantly tamper, taking out the battery and complaining that it was uncomfortable or wasn't working properly. She would often test the patience of each and every carer and nurse in the home!

As a result, this would affect her ability to listen and hear music. Nevertheless, Dorothea participated in most music sessions. She would waste little time in telling me exactly which music she liked and disliked and for how long I should play for her. She would get angry and frustrated if she could not hear the music properly but would not listen when a carer would explain to her that constantly tampering with the hearing aid was not helping. However, she loved the sound of the harp and would come out with comments such as, 'It's beautiful. Play me one more.'

Dorothea was very strict and took no nonsense, but she also possessed a softer, more vulnerable side. I'd noticed her one morning standing by the nurse's hub, asking many questions and demanding 'proper answers' before the nurse finally managed to get on her way and carry out her daily morning rounds. When I saw Dorothea a little while later, she was sitting in a chair outside the nurse's hub with her head in her hands, in obvious distress and bewilderment. I kneeled down next to Dorothea so she could hear me and asked her what seemed to be worrying her.

'Something terrible has happened', she said. 'They say I'm …' She paused for a moment; her expression incredulous. She started again. 'They say I'm … NINETY-EIGHT!' She looked at me in desperation for a moment before continuing. 'But you see, I must have lost my mother *and* my father …' She paused. 'And I think I may have lost my brother. And even my husband. They're all gone. All dead!' With a look of abject defeat etched across her pale face, she conceded. 'This is terrible. I've lost so much!' She looked down at her hands with tears filling her eyes; then said, her voice shaking, 'I don't remember losing them.'

How does one console somebody weighed down by all this grief? Dorothea always wanted answers. She tried to comprehend what was happening to her, to make sense of it all. This was why she would persistently plague the nurses with endless questions. She wanted to know what was causing her so much distress. Consoling her was not going to be enough. I would have to try and reason with her somehow and try to convince her to come to terms with the realisation that her entire family had passed away over time and somehow disentangle the jumbled sequence of past events that no longer made sense to her.

I took both her hands in mine and looked at her face-to-face.

'Dorothea, I know this must be terrible for you, but I think you may already know that your family has passed away and that sometimes you forget. You will have grieved for each and every one of them at a certain time in your life. You've lived a long and full life, which I love hearing about during our little chats together'. I talked gently to her, and she seemed to listen and comprehend what I was saying. We went to make a cup of tea together and then went to her bedroom to have a look through her photo album. She started chatting about the stories behind the pictures. Reminiscing seemed to make her feel better, at least for the time being.

A few weeks before Dorothea's death at ninety-nine years old, we had a short one-to-one session with the little Celtic harp in her room. After playing a few of her favourite melodies, she suddenly raised her hand and said, 'Stop, please! It's too poignant'. This, once again, revealed a softer and more vulnerable side to a strong, capable and determined woman who had lived a whole lifetime, drinking deeply and richly from life's many experiences. Despite her dementia, Dorothea's memory retained a trace of some of the good times she had experienced, which provided comfort for her in times of need.

*****

Elena was a sweet-natured lady, kind and lovely. She had dementia and Parkinson's disease. Her family informed me that she loved to sing before the dementia progressed but would still occasionally sing favourites with a beautiful voice in the care home, such as 'Crazy' by Patsy Cline and 'The Tennessee Waltz' by Patti Page.

Elena was able to attend the sessions in the music room and would engage well at times. But there were moments when she would close her eyes and simply shut down, away from the world around her. As her dementia progressed, this would happen more and more often, and no amount of reassurance, coaxing or kind words would make her open her eyes and reconnect. It felt to me as if she was simply trying to stop the pain of her situation. I had witnessed her cry so desperately – it was heart-wrenching to watch – and all one could do during those desperate times was to hold her in one's arms and comfort her.

Elena had led a full life and had travelled the world. Her photo albums were full of photographs of her travels with her husband to exotic places in the Far East. The photos showed a youthful looking Elena smiling into the lens of the camera, living her life to the full, thankfully oblivious to what lay ahead of her later in life. Elena did not always recognise her husband when he visited, but when she did, she would look at him with total love and devotion in her eyes. During those times of recognition, it would break her heart to see him leave, and she would retreat further into herself for hours after he'd left.

Elena loved shoes and handbags, and her husband informed me that she had dozens of them at home. Sometimes, Elena and I would put some of her favourite music to play in the background, and then we would sit together looking at hundreds of different styles of shoes and handbags on my iPad, with Elena pointing and occasionally commenting on the ones she took a fancy to. Yes, there were good days and bad days. As poet Dylan Thomas put it, these residents' grief often flowed because of 'the rift of unremembered skies and snows', and of many other memories, now long forgotten.

5. The Silent Guitarist

Don used to be a drayman. Tall and strong, he would sit in his special chair in a corner of the lounge. This provided him with an ideal vantage point, allowing him to see the comings and goings of the day – the staff changing their shifts, delivery lorries arriving with goods for the kitchen, friends and families arriving to visit loved ones, and so on. I would wave at Don through the window when I arrived for work in the morning, and he would return this with a huge, broad smile.

In his youth, Don used to play guitar in a band with some friends, and so when one of the carers offered to bring an old, unused acoustic guitar to work, I immediately thought of taking it to Don. I was curious to find out how much he might remember. When presented with the guitar, Don immediately curled the fingers of his left hand around the fretboard to play a series of familiar chord patterns.

However, he could not actually make himself strum these chords with his right hand. He obviously remembered chord patterns and sequences – the hard part – but could not remember the easy bit: how to strum. It was as if the right side of the brain, which controls the left side of the body, seemed to work, but the left side of the brain, controlling the right side of the body, failed to flex Don's muscle memory to enable him to strum those chords and bring them back to life. Perched on Don's knees, the guitar remained poignantly silent – yet another sign of dementia's disruptive and destructive effects.

Don's favourite artist was Elvis Presley and he would often sing along to 'I Can't Help Falling in Love With You'. However, he would often get upset when singing this particular song. A little while later I was told by his wife that this song had always been special to them. One could see quite clearly that Don and his wife still loved each other very much. Even though she wasn't in the best of health herself, she would travel by taxi on a hundred-mile round-trip to visit her husband every week. Don had originally come to the care home as a temporary arrangement only, while his wife and daughter found somewhere that catered for his needs while also being closer to their home.

However, it appeared that Don had settled in well in this particular place, and his wife and daughter concluded that it was probably in his best interests for him to stay where he was. While they had to put up with the long-distance travel, Don's welfare was ultimately more important.

But there were times when Don, like many other residents – and indeed like most of us – would get irritable and impatient. He would lash out and shout at the world in words that made no sense, although the expression on his face spoke volumes. Being such a big, strong man, his behaviour could become quite frightening to witness. On one occasion, while noticing the carers trying desperately to placate Don, the well-known lines from another Dylan Thomas poem came to my mind:

> *Do not go gentle into that good night,*
> *Old age should burn and rave at close of day;*
> *Rage, rage against the dying of the light.*

The last line seemed especially poignant. Dementia's cruel power would often force people like Don to 'Rage, rage against the dying of the light'. He, for one, was not going gently into that good night. Yet, as well as being a gentleman, Don was also a 'gentle man' at heart. He would sit by the window gazing out with the sun upon his face. Many residents, before their dementia set in, would often be outdoors because of their profession, or simply because they enjoyed being outdoors. They would go for walks, do a bit of gardening, or maybe play a game of golf.

I would often try to make time during the day to take Don out in his wheelchair. He loved to feel the wind on his face. Released momentarily from the confines of the care home, I loved to see the beaming smile on his face as soon as we went out through the main door. He would look up towards the sun – leaning forward in the wheelchair to breathe in huge gulps of fresh air – and a wonderful smile would become permanently fixed on his face the whole time we were outside.

Once, I took a photo of him wrapped up in his coat, smiling in the autumn sunshine. His wife later thanked me for taking him out, telling me ruefully, 'I don't think he ever went out in the two years he was at his previous care home'. Very soon, Don understood that when I popped my head around the door of his lounge to say 'Hello', there was a good chance we were going to have some music, or – weather permitting – we would be going out for a stroll.

A huge smile would spread across his face as he reached his arms out towards me. There were times when I was just 'looking in' on my way to see somebody else and he would start crying loudly when I turned to leave! I would then have to try to reassure him, promising him that I would return. It was difficult to just bring him with me as he needed two carers to move him from his chair to a wheelchair, which all took time, effort and manpower. This could become quite frustrating for all concerned as it would have been good to just be able to 'up and go' like some other residents were able to do.

It is so important that care homes try as best they can to provide quality events for their residents. Going that extra mile makes so much difference, even if it takes more time and effort and may end up costing more money. The buzzword in recent years has been *enrichment*: how best to enrich the lives of PWD. Clearly this can be done through music and other art forms. But what kind of music? What kind of art? How can we enrich the lives of *all* the residents while also catering for each one's particular tastes and needs?

My own view is that, while it's important to have fun and keep things light-hearted, we should generally avoid the *Hi-de-Hi!* 'holiday camp'-style entertainment. Regrettably, this kind of entertainment is the norm in some care homes.

Residents deserve better than a staple diet of bingo, karaoke, or swatting balloons around a room. Of course, this kind of entertainment is better than no provision at all, with daytime TV the lowest form of all in my view, used in some homes as an 'opiate for the masses'. Just in the same way that a varied diet of food is good, a varied diet of entertainment is also needed. In fact, sometimes light entertainment is preferred by some residents and should therefore be respected and represented.

I soon found that many residents enjoyed Elvis's songs, unsurprising given that many of them grew up during the height of the great singer's powers during the late 1950s and early 60s. I relented to my own personal misgivings by organising a visit by a locally based Elvis impersonator to come and entertain the residents. I had previously managed to create some arrangements of Elvis's love songs on the harp for the singalong sessions, and we'd played some of his livelier songs during some of the 'Music and Movement' sessions at the home,[15] but that was the extent of Elvis for me as far as I was concerned.

15   For more on the 'Music and Movement' sessions, see Chapter 11.

I didn't have to do much reminding about the event, as many residents (and indeed the carers themselves) were looking forward excitedly to the day when 'Elvis' was arriving. Don was one of the attendees, as were all the other Elvis fans. There was a definite buzz around the care home that morning. Every possible space was taken in the music room, and the hallway outside the music room was also crammed with carers and other staff, equally eager to experience a piece of the action!

After much anticipation, in walked 'Elvis', dressed in all his sequined finery. I must admit, he had quite a presence about him, and everybody seemed to enjoy his performance. Maybe some of the residents actually thought that this was the man himself, returned from the dead! This particular 'Elvis' was a chaplain at the local general hospital and was therefore very much used to working with people in a very special way and in similar circumstances. He connected well with the residents and had been briefed about those residents who were lifelong fans of the 'King'. He approached Don and sang one of his favourite songs for him. Don watched him, transfixed, with tears in his eyes, smiling throughout.

There was plenty of singing to be heard, and it was good to see the carers singing along with the residents. This was a moment of much-needed respite for many of them – temporarily released from their day-to-day duties – as everyone's focus was now on the singer in the shining suit shaking his pelvis to 'Hound Dog'. Had he lived, Elvis would have been around the same age as many of these residents. His music defined their era and their youth. His songs provided the soundtrack to the giddy flush and bloom of adolescence and the birth of rock 'n' roll that many of these residents had witnessed and experienced at first hand.

Plenty of photos were taken to show the families of the residents how much everybody seemed to have enjoyed themselves that morning. Needless to say, Elvis was a huge hit with all who attended, including me, and the 'King' was to return again to the care home by popular demand!

6. Singing Together in a Group

'What cannot be said in our day is sung.'

I conduct many group sessions, where the attendance can vary from between ten to around thirty residents. A little background on the benefits of singing in a group is needed here, as this is a major part of the work I do as a musician.

The tendency amongst people who have been diagnosed with any form of dementia is to slowly retreat from their community and social activities because they don't want to be seen as being forgetful and confused.

Singing in a group is a social activity that brings people who find themselves in a similar situation closer together. It can boost emotional wellbeing and fuel self-respect. It can relieve tension, depression, confusion and anxiety. Furthermore, recent studies have shown that active participation through singing can also be an effective means of expression.

Terrence Hays and Victor Minichiello's research in Australia has studied the significance of music on the lives of the elderly, including some PWD. Their work has highlighted the importance of music for individuals' self-respect, their wellbeing, their ability to connect with others in order to avoid feelings of loneliness. They conclude that, 'Music is an important part of the lives of people because it is through music that they can come to know and reflect upon their own personhood.'[16]

In one part of her research dissertation, which focuses on therapy with persons in advanced stages of dementia in Denmark, music therapist Hanne Mette Ochsner Ridder discusses a short questionnaire that was distributed in a seminar held for carers of the elderly. The purpose of this short questionnaire was to discover which musical activities appealed most to them (including some with dementia), such as listening to music, combining music with movement, or playing instruments. The questionnaire showed that singing along together was the most popular musical activity. Ridder explains:

> *The elderly generation in Denmark has grown up in a very strong song tradition where people would sing when they met for celebrations, political meetings, and cultural events. This might be a significant reason still to use songs when people come together.*[17]

---

16 T. Hays, V. Minichiello, 'The meaning of music in the lives of older people: a qualitative study', *Psychology of Music*, 33 (2005), p. 440.

17 Hanne Mette Ochsner Ridder, 'Singing dialogue, Music therapy with persons in advanced stages of dementia. A case study research design', Ph.D thesis, Ålborg University, Institute for Music and Music Therapy (2003), p. 38.

Of course, this is also true in the case of many other countries. Brynjulf Stige, a professor at the University of Bergen, conducted observations over a period of several weeks on group singing with an elderly choir in Norway to support his research work. Stige immediately saw how important being part of a choir could be for the elderly as it created a community of caring for one another between its members.[18]

The Welsh have a very strong tradition of singing together too, for many generations – be it through congregational hymn-singing in chapels or informal get-togethers in pubs, male voice choirs of the coal pits and slate communities, collective singing before and during rugby matches, as well as the strong tradition of the Eisteddfod.[19] Even in the case of elderly people who are not Welsh and may have moved to Wales to retire, they are mostly aware of the strong Welsh tradition of singing together.

Over the years, my repertoire of songs has grown to fill several files with various songs of all kinds. From hymns to rock 'n' roll, from songs written during the First World War to popular Beatles hits, from old traditional Celtic tunes to classical songs – all of them reflect the diverse range of musical tastes, preferences and interests of the many residents I have been in contact with over time. Indeed, I have been fortunate enough to have learned so

18 Brynjulf Stige, 'Caring for Music: The Senior Choir in Sandane Norway', in Stige, Ansdell, Elefant and Pavlicevic (ed.), *Where Music Helps: Community Music Therapy in Action and Reflection* (Ashgate, 2010), pp. 245–274.
19 For more on this, see Gareth Williams, *Valleys of Song: Music and Society in Wales, 1840–1914* (University of Wales Press, 1998).

many interesting songs over the years due to the need to satisfy residents' specific musical requests!

I was once requested to sing Rod Stuart's 'I am Sailing' by one of the residents. As I sang the song, accompanying myself on the piano, it suddenly struck me how poignant the words were to a couple of the verses:

> *We are sailing, we are sailing,*
> *Home again, 'cross the sea;*
> *We are sailing, stormy waters,*
> *To be near you, to be free.*

> *Can you hear me, can you hear me,*
> *Through the dark night, far away;*
> *I am dying, forever crying,*
> *To be with you, who can say.*

As the residents all sang these words, it did indeed feel as if each one of them was sailing stormy waters, trying to get home to be near their loved ones, free from the confusion and destruction of dementia.

On a more upbeat note, several lighter songs have also proved very popular in group sessions, so-called 'sequence' songs, such as the Welsh folksong '*Cyfri'r Geifr*' ('Counting the Goats'). This traditional rural song is about milking the goats, with each verse listing a different coloured goat in need of milking. As the sequence of verses extends ('a white goat', 'a red goat', 'a black goat', 'a pink goat', and so on), it becomes increasingly challenging to remember all the different coloured goats in the correct order. It nevertheless fails to surprise me how well many of the residents manage to remember the colour sequence, with music again providing the support.

Round songs are also popular and can be fun, such as 'Frère Jacques' and 'Row, Row, Row Your Boat'. Of course, songs such as these are not only enjoyable to sing but they also exercise the mind. In a fun way and through music, they test one's memory. Residents have to focus harder when performing such songs. It always amazes me and is quite remarkable how a certain sequence in a song can be remembered if the words are hung on to a familiar melody, or how residents can focus on a certain part of a song while others around them are singing a different part, as in 'Row, Row, Row Your Boat'.

Many people with dementia often seem to lose their inhibitions when it comes to singing. Unlike many elderly people who feel somewhat self-conscious that their singing voice has deteriorated, quite a number of PWD no longer seem to care what their voices sound like, or whether they are singing in tune or not. As this is not often an issue when they are singing, they will sing without caring what anybody thinks!

Some residents will state that although they plan on attending a singing session they won't be joining in the singing, yet they will almost always end up singing in the end. There are other residents who will chose not to participate actively by singing but will nevertheless

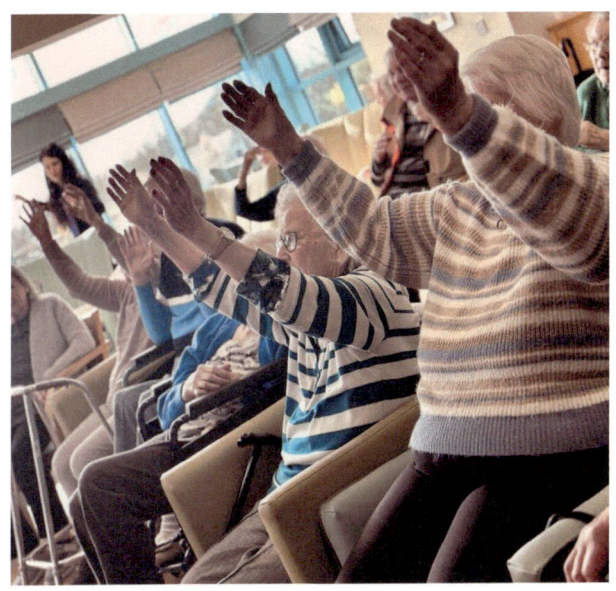

enjoy the session through passive participation only. It is important that the choice of whether to actively participate or not is always respected.

One lady who regularly attended group singing sessions would feel the overwhelming need to conduct the singing with her arms. She would wave them about, motivating her own singing – and others around her – onwards. Another lady would start to sing the minute she entered the music room, even before the music had begun! If I was simply by my desk catching up with some administrative work and she could see that I was in the music room, she'd come in and start singing: a direct connection was established in her mind between the music room, my work and the singing sessions held there.

At one of the main care homes where I worked, we would sing together so frequently that when, for example, a choir would visit, or I would take some residents with me to a local concert, the ones who regularly attended my group sessions would immediately burst into song with the singers on stage! For the residents, this seemed a perfectly normal thing to do, and I loved and admired them for doing so.

During these times, I felt that we were a team – wonderful people singing from their hearts because they felt like it, no matter whether it was the 'done' thing or not. It was heart-warming to see members of a choir, a conductor or accompanist smile as they saw and heard a group of people singing along, losing themselves in the music, smiling and clearly enjoying themselves. The expectations of how to conduct oneself in society had vanished. If you felt like singing along to a choir, then what was there to stop you? Certainly not dementia!

This is why raising awareness of dementia and what to expect from PWD should be shared with people of all ages and in all strands of society. Schemes like 'Dementia Friends' by the Alzheimer's Society – where dementia awareness courses are given to businesses, organisations and individuals – are becoming increasingly widespread in communities, as are making villages, towns, and even cities, dementia-friendly zones.

In many theatres and cinemas, there are special dementia-friendly performances and viewings. In these performances, performers and their companies are taught to be more tolerant to PWD, who may call out or walk about during performances. Cinema screenings are shown with subtle lighting as opposed to complete darkness and the volume turned down from its usual loud setting. These are all excellent schemes which serve to 'normalise' dementia in society.

Many students, documentary makers, news reporters, visiting dignitaries, theatre companies, radio producers, university researchers – not to mention individuals on work experience – have shadowed me during my work, and it is during group sessions such as those mentioned above that they gain the best experience of the effects of music on people who live with dementia. Visiting parties are often quite taken aback by residents' abilities to sing quite effortlessly, especially if they have tried to have a conversation with some of the residents beforehand and found very little conversation or communication forthcoming.

It became apparent to me during such sessions that many residents with various forms of dementia at different stages of the disease could even learn new songs with simple words and melodies. This would make a great opportunity for further research – the fact that many people who have a disease that disables their short-term memory can, in fact, not only remember songs they already know but also learn some new songs too. And perhaps even more importantly, they can remember them!

Another interesting fact is that the lift at one of the larger care homes where I have worked, which takes the residents directly into the music room, will inform those travelling in it in both English and Welsh, that the 'Lift is going up / *Lifft yn mynd i fyny*', before reaching the 'First floor / *Llawr cyntaf*'. On immediately entering the lift, some residents will announce these statements in both languages, regardless of whether they speak both languages: they will remember the tone of voice, the context, and the exact statement.

We often have a laugh about it at the time, but this is an example of residents remembering something from their day-to-day lives at the care home – something they have picked up and remembered from the very recent past, not something deeply embedded in their memories from early childhood. I am convinced that their ability to recall short-term phrases such as 'Lift is going up' is linked to the fact that they are coming to the music room to sing. They are remembering. Or perhaps, more accurately, as they get ready for the music session, they are remembering to remember. I firmly believe that music sessions have a positive knock-on effect on residents' surrounding circumstances and environment.

As noted already in this book's introduction, Robin Rio has discussed the benefits of music when remembering and learning new things. Group sessions can provide excellent opportunities by introducing new songs to the repertoire, or through offering translations of songs where the PWD might be familiar with the tune but not with the words. Rio explains:

Music itself is patterned and organised sounds, much more organised than typical speech. Remembering a conversation may be hard, but remembering a series of organised notes or a poem is much easier.[20]

When I'm sometimes asked to give a talk or presentation about my work, I usually start each talk with a short quote – repeated a couple of times – which I then encourage the audience to recite it aloud with me. I will then proceed to follow the quote by getting the audience to sing a short song with me, which is also repeated a couple of times. Both the quote and song will be unfamiliar to the audience. An hour or so later, when I have concluded my talk or presentation and all subsequent questions answered and discussed, I return to the quote given at the beginning and ask the audience to recite it back to me.

At this point there will always be some embarrassed faces with some audience members shuffling uneasily in their chairs. Most will struggle to remember the quote in its entirety. Some will recollect fragments of it, but on the whole, large parts of the quote will be forgotten. However, when I ask the same people to sing the short, unfamiliar song heard at the beginning back to me, the success rate will be much higher. If nothing else, this little demonstration proves just how effective music can be in relation to memory.

20   Robin Rio, *Connecting Through Music with People with Dementia: A Guide for Caregivers* (London, 2009), p. 92.

7. The Piano and Other Instruments

One day, with much excitement on my part, a baby grand piano was delivered to the music room on the first floor of one of the care homes where I worked. The piano had arrived at the home on the same afternoon as a wonderfully eccentric new resident called Beatrice. I was told that Beatrice loved music, especially classical music. How serendipitous that Beatrice and the piano should arrive on the same day!

A couple of weeks later, Beatrice's son visited the home to see how his mother was settling in. Talking in the care home manager's office over a cup of coffee, we started off by chatting about the arrival of the baby grand piano, but soon enough he had moved on to enquire about how we had taken his mother upstairs to the music room. Still thinking that we were discussing the baby grand, I explained: 'Well, we simply unscrewed her legs and turned her on her side. She fitted quite nicely into the lift that way...'

Somehow managing to ignore the look of utter incredulity and horror upon Beatrice's son's face, I proceeded to tell him, 'Oh, don't worry, she's quite all right, you know. We simply screwed her legs back on. She'll settle after a few weeks if left alone without too much movement.' It was only when I saw the care home manager's mouth hanging open in incredulity from the corner of my eye that I realised we were both talking about two entirely different things…

Yes, Beatrice loved classical music, and so when a wonderful string quartet agreed to do a session for us as part of their work as a quartet-in-residence at a nearby University, I immediately thought of bringing Beatrice to the lunchtime soirée knowing she would appreciate their wonderful playing and recognise the repertoire well.

However, just as the quartet were tuning their instruments prior to playing the first piece in the concert, Beatrice announced loudly to the whole room: 'They're dreadful! Absolutely dreadful! Take me out of here *immediately*!' No amount of pleading or persuading would convince Beatrice otherwise. The fact that the quartet were only tuning meant little to Beatrice. No reassurance or reasoning was enough to placate Beatrice, and she was duly wheeled away from the music room back to the lounge. Needless to say, I was disappointed that Beatrice did not get to hear the quartet, who gave a wonderful concert while Beatrice sat in the lounge, cup of Earl Grey tea in hand, enjoying a piece of cake.

I'm glad to say that after this unpromising beginning, Beatrice did manage to attend and enjoy many concerts at the home, from beginning to end. I also managed to conduct some lovely one-to-one music sessions with her, and when the music stopped she would sometimes pause and say, 'That's lovely', or 'Very nice'. But after a short while, she would shut her eyes and say, 'That's enough now'.

While all residents are unique in their own special way, some truly shine out, and for various reasons Beatrice was one of them. She had lived an interesting, colourful and eventful life, travelling all over the world, and I felt privileged to have shared part of her life with her, even if it was just the final chapter.

As I had discovered at the classical music concert some months previously, Beatrice could be cuttingly direct and honest. But this was a characteristic I admired in her. I'll never forget her son coming up to me the day after she passed away. He'd been by her side constantly during her final days and hours, only leaving briefly every so often to catch a bit of fresh air.

Just before what turned out to be his final visit, Beatrice looked at her son and said candidly, 'Don't go wasting your time crying over me.' She died a couple of hours later. It was as if she'd waited for him to leave the room before leaving the world herself. Beatrice knew that her days were numbered, and she had made her peace with life. I was honoured when the family asked me to play her favourite hymn, 'Gwahoddiad', at her funeral.

A couple of years after Beatrice passed away, a gentleman called Malcolm arrived at the same care home. His family noted that he preferred to spend time in his bedroom in peace rather than being in the lounge with the other male residents, and he would not appreciate joining any of the many group sessions offered. One always had to respect the family's wishes, of course. Maybe the family's request related to the fact that the lounge in which Malcolm lived could be quite noisy with some residents often calling out loudly.

Still, it was a shame to see Malcolm constantly in his room, although he appeared fairly content, listening much of the time to classical music on the radio. As I was arriving to work one morning, one of the carers from Malcolm's lounge approached me and said that while listening to a piano concerto on the radio, she'd noticed him simulating the sounds and motion of the piece with his hands on his knees. I was aware that Malcolm enjoyed music, but respected his privacy, so I thought I would take him up to the music room after the group session finished – just him and me – and we could sit together by the piano and then see how things might go.

When Malcolm first saw the piano, he was obviously delighted and exclaimed, 'A piano! How wonderful!' I wheeled him right up to the keys and placed his feet gently near the pedals. This was the start of some lovely one-to-one sessions where Malcolm explained – gesturing with his hand – how he used to stand just knee high to his father, watching him play the piano.

It was obvious from the start that, like his father, Malcolm also played the piano. His hands travelled along the keys, picking out some chords that still remained intact in his memory. He would often get frustrated when he failed to remember how to play melodies and chords but would carry on the melody by humming the tune and occasionally picking out the melody again on the piano. He didn't seem to mind me joining him on the piano while he tried to figure out a familiar melody and map it out on the keys, but I always let him take the lead. Despite some frustrations, Malcolm continued to enjoy each session, which usually ended with him requesting that I 'play something for me now!'

*****

Like Malcolm, there are many residents who used to play the piano, and I'd often bring those residents to the music room for one-to-one sessions which might involve a chat about the piano pieces they'd enjoyed playing once upon a time. I'd gently encourage them to run their fingers across the keys to see if they could remember parts of a piano piece that they'd used to play. I'd also play some well-known pieces to see if the residents could identify them.

Elliot, a retired medical professor, used to play piano. I was informed by Elliot's family that, in his youth, he succeeded in his exams all the way up to Grade 8. When

I brought Elliot to the piano, he talked to me about what I'd already been told by his family – that he had owned an ebony upright Steinway piano. Elliot went on to explain that his piano was one of the last consignment of pianos delivered to Coventry just before the onset of the Second World War. It never ceases to bring me joy – the way music can be such a fantastic mode to open up avenues of communication, thereby reaching the person behind the dementia.

Elliot would also love listening to the harp, but music often made him become very emotional. He would comment that he loved the sound of the harp, but once admitted, 'It makes me cry'. Some of the music we played brought back vivid memories of the war, and without prompting he would say, 'They shot down his plane. They shot down my friend's plane!' These were obviously painful memories for Elliot. The Welsh hymn, 'Calon Lân' (Pure Heart) reminded him of his friend. He explained that his lost friends' 'aunt' would sing it to him as a child.

Elliot's day-to-day existence was in a purpose-made chair. His movement was increasingly restricted as his body became frailer and more twisted. He could not reach out very well and therefore it was very difficult for him to put his fingers on the piano's keys or on the harp's strings. Instead, I would bring the little Celtic harp within touching distance of Elliot so that he could feel the vibrations coming from the instrument's sound box when striking a chord or playing a glissando. This way of doing things seemed to work as he found it quite enjoyable.

Elliot was certainly more alert during most singing sessions and especially during the one-to-one sessions. He would also be very lucid after we played some music, and although he could become very emotional and tearful at times during the sessions, Elliot seemed happier at the end of the session, as if the whole experience had been a catharsis for him.

*****

Apart from the piano, the main instrument I have used over the years as part of my work has been a little Celtic harp. Unlike the piano or pedal harp, the Celtic harp is easily transportable. This means I can carry it around with me when I work, visiting residents in their rooms for one-to-one sessions if they are too frail or unwell to attend sessions in the music room. Furthermore, the Celtic harp is small and light enough to place on a resident's knee so he or she can run their fingers along the strings. As shown with Elliot, allowing residents to engage with musical sounds is really important. This tactile connection with sound itself opens avenues of communication through music.

I also use a concert, pedal harp which is much bigger and heavier. (It has 47 strings as opposed to 26 strings on my Celtic harp.) The concert harp has a fuller, richer sound but is much less portable and therefore gets used less. However, it is a beautiful instrument, and most people enjoy listening to the sound of the harp. The harp itself is a very therapeutic instrument and can be used just to play quiet, relaxing music to a resident that may be particularly unwell or going through a restless time. Its therapeutic qualities extend at least as far back as the Old Testament, when David soothed Saul with his harp: 'David would play his harp. Saul would relax and feel better, and the evil spirit would go away.'[21]

This was certainly the case with many residents I came to know. Nicholas enjoyed listening to music played on the harp and to my singing. It seemed to have the desired effect, which was to calm Nicholas down when he was feeling restless or anxious. He became more relaxed and would sometimes dose off during the session.

During one of my one-to-one sessions with Nicholas, I brought the little harp within touching distance to him, then something quite extraordinary and unexpected happened. Nicholas gradually ran one of his hands down the strings of the harp. After reaching and plucking the lowest string, he would then cup his hands, bringing them shakily to his mouth, as if 'drinking' the notes that he had just played.

Why was Nicholas doing this? What made him want to cup his hands and bring them to his mouth? It was as if he was trying to 'capture' the sound of the strings at the base of the instrument and somehow trying to ingest and imbibe those sounds. Nicholas's condition meant that he often hallucinated. When he brushed the harp's strings with his hands, was he 'seeing' something else, perhaps in his mind's eye? There were times when I wasn't sure if I was getting

---

21   Samuel 16:23.

through to Nicholas, but after hearing a song or piece of music on the harp he seemed more relaxed, more 'centred' somehow. He would sit with his eyes closed, and comment quietly, 'That's beautiful', or 'That's nice, one more...'

Nicholas's wife would visit at some point nearly every day. I asked whether she would mind telling me when she started noticing that things weren't quite right with her husband. She said that, in hindsight, she had suspected

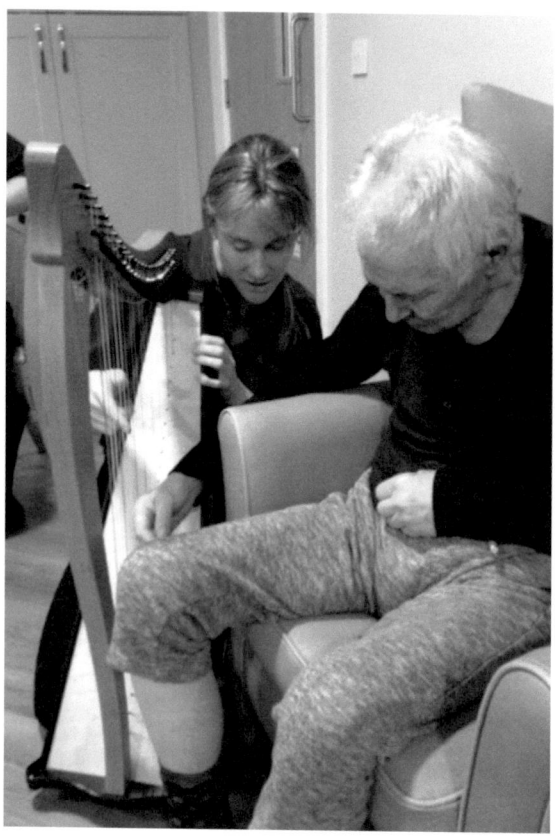

that all was not well probably a couple of years before the diagnosis, but tried to dismiss the warning signs at first. Looking back, she recognised that she had not wanted to face up to the fact that something serious was going on with Nicholas. But she knew she could not live in denial for too long and soon enough everything came to a head one day during a family meal at a restaurant.

Nicholas had left the table to go to the gents room. After a while, when his wife started wondering where he was, a waitress came to the table to tell her that her husband seemed to be distressed and was standing near the door to the toilet. Having hurried over to investigate what was going on, it turned out that Nicholas simply could not negotiate himself through the two sets of doors leading in and out of the toilet. He had become very confused and upset. Negotiating oneself through a few sets of doors – a relatively straightforward procedure for most of us – can become a major challenge for someone even in the early stages of dementia. They can become increasingly disorientated by various entries, exits and stairs and how to navigate them.

This unfortunate episode became a catalyst for Nicholas's wife and family. It was now time to face up to the truth and take him to see a doctor for a diagnosis. As I write this chapter, I recall Nicholas's wife once mentioning that on more than one occasion he had fallen and banged his head badly. She couldn't help thinking that this injury may have caused – or at least contributed to – Nicholas's dementia. It has become known now that head injuries, particularly persistent head injuries, can cause a certain form of dementia.[22] Research is now being carried out to try to ascertain and better understand the link between persistent head injuries and dementia.

*****

The piano is the most appropriate instrument for using during large group sessions and for playing more up-beat songs. It's also useful for conducting one-to-ones with residents who used to play the piano or who have a particular affinity with the instrument. The harp is the perfect therapeutic instrument, however, and is loved by most people.

However, the instrument that I use by far the most often, and which is the most portable of all, is my voice. Singing gently to a confused and lonely resident can be soothing, if you know when it is appropriate to do so. One can sing with somebody just by walking through the gardens or when going for a drive in the car. Singing brings people together more than just through listening to music.

I also have a large box of professional percussion instruments which I sometimes draw upon during music sessions. These include chimes, wood blocks, tambourines, maracas, castanets, various drums, xylophone, bells,

22 This is called Chronic Traumatic Encephalopathy (CTE). It's a progressive degenerative disease of the brain found commonly in boxers. It has also been linked with professional football players active during the 1950s and 60s, repeatedly heading footballs that were much heavier than those that are used today.

cymbals, and a rain stick. The box also includes an ocean drum, which is not an instrument that is struck (as its name suggests), but rather an instrument that you move gently from side to side. It is filled with many small ball-bearings that can be seen inside the drum. When moved gently and continuously, the noise of all the ball-bearings moving inside creates the sound of the ocean's waves breaking upon the shore.

Percussion instruments are used mainly by the residents, with the help of the carers if needed. I've collected many photographs of residents' happy faces over the years, enjoying themselves with percussion instruments during a music session. They certainly can add an element of fun to the sessions, and they can also help with movement and coordination.[23]

Many of these percussion instruments are used during certain songs, for example, to add a beat or an effect. I have used the ocean drum during a rendition of 'The Skye Boat Song', for example. I have also used percussion instruments during the traditional Irish song 'Molly Malone' (or 'Cockles and Mussels'), where I share out maracas among some residents to represent the 'cockles', and then tambourines for others to represent the 'mussels'. Once we'd come to the part where we'd sing 'Singing Cockles and Mussels / Alive, alive, Oh!' the residents would be encouraged to shake their respective instruments accordingly! Active and creative participation is an essential feature of music-making, and residents are always encouraged to join in.

---

23   Music and Movement will be discussed a little later in this book.

8. Concerts

A concert is about to begin featuring a highly regarded and well-established soloist performing well-known repertoire. Just as he is about to sing the opening song in the program there comes a remark from the front of the audience: 'I can't believe we're missing *Coronation Street* for this!'

The performance progresses. Suddenly, a slipper is thrown towards the soloist. Thankfully he seems unperturbed by the furry missile which lands with a flop beside his feet. Just as the applause dies down at the conclusion of the final piece in the recital, a voice is heard at the back, shouting, 'Where's my teeth? Has anybody seen my teeth?'

As you've probably gathered, this is no ordinary concert. And this is no ordinary audience either. The concert took place in the music room of a large dementia care centre. It must be said that the majority of the residents fully enjoyed this particular concert, but you just never know what kind of reaction you may get from the very special audience that attends such concerts.

As a resident musician in a large dementia care centre, my role was not only to conduct music sessions and organise one-to-one sessions with residents but also to connect with outside organisations, such as local primary and secondary schools, the music faculty at the nearby University, performers giving concerts at the local arts centre, in addition to choirs, quartets, vocal groups, folk singers and other musicians.

My role was to provide wide, varied and quality musical experiences for the residents of the home. On occasion this would involve linking up with professional organisations such as the Royal Liverpool Philharmonic Orchestra or Welsh National Opera when they visited North Wales as part of one of their tours. A couple of chorus members from the opera company or a few musicians from the orchestra would turn up and perform a small concert for the residents, thus ensuring that the quality of the performances were of a very high standard.

Before being admitted into the care home, many residents had regularly frequented productions and performances at theatres, concert halls and opera houses. It was therefore extremely important to continue to provide similar experiences for them in this way.

However, many of the most amusing incidents over the years have often occurred during such concerts. Once, a world-renowned soprano had visited the nearby University's Arts Centre for a week-long residency. The residency involved an outreach community-based program, which meant that she would visit the dementia care centre where I worked to give a short lunchtime concert. The soprano duly arrived at the appointed time with a wonderfully accomplished accompanist on piano. There was a palpable sense of anticipation in the air as residents were gradually brought into the music room for the start of the event.

Clearly wishing to create a striking impression from the outset, the soprano immediately launched into a powerful and dramatic aria from a Verdi opera. After a series of solemn and serious chords on the piano, she started to sing – her voice deep, low and resonant at the beginning. Then her voice started rising, soaring ever higher and higher in pitch and becoming louder and louder. The walls, windows and very foundations of the music room started to shake to her thunderous voice, until the aria reached a resounding and shuddering climax, followed by deafening silence.

Transfixed to the singer up until this point, I suddenly looked over to the audience to see most of the residents with their fingers plugged firmly in their ears! Many of them assumed this posture throughout the performance. A second song followed in much the same vein. This time a gentleman resident at the back could be heard shouting, 'Too loud!' Then, after a brief while, 'It's still too loud!'

During the introduction to the third song, the soprano – a woman of ample girth and proportions, who was probably in her mid-sixties – took a long intake of breath in preparation for the lengthy, sustained opening note. One of the residents could be heard to quip quite loudly, 'Good God! She can't possibly be pregnant at that age, can she?'

While a seasoned performer will rarely become perturbed by such instances, many carers and family members will sit there, red faced with embarrassment. Before the start of a concert at the care home, I will always take visiting performers to one side and discretely explain to them that they should take all reactions and comments in good faith and humour. They should not feel offended by any responses or take any comments personally. Many are often already fully aware of the kinds of possible reactions, having performed at such places many times before.

The enrichment value far outweighs any possible humiliation a performer might feel, and most of the time experienced performers will accept it as being part-and-parcel of the whole experience. In fact, they often enjoy themselves as much, if not more, when performing in such situations, than they might do in the more formal setting of a concert hall or opera house.

Just as the residents often lose their inhibitions in a concert situation, expressing out loudly what they actually think, likewise performers will let go of their inhibitions too. They can let go of the stiff and formal concert-hall etiquette that they are used to following from one week to the next. I sometimes imagine that perhaps this more relaxed setting was how classical concerts would have been like in the age of Mozart and Beethoven, with performances taking place in less formal surroundings and audiences being far more direct and vocal in their responses. One can imagine someone in the audience shouting out during the premiere of one of Beethoven's symphonies, 'It's still too loud!'

While many amusing moments have occurred in such concerts, there have been very many more poignant moments. Malcolm, who was introduced to the reader in an earlier chapter, would conduct the visiting soprano with his hands while still seated – his arms waving about and reaching up to prod the air with his fingers as she scaled up to the high notes.

During a rendition of Schubert's 'Trout', Malcolm would mimic the piano's gliding, agile accompaniment with his fingers bouncing on his knees. I could see that he became very emotional during one beautifully sung aria. After the concert ended, he said to me, 'She made my eyes rain.' Residents would often come out with honest, beautiful and heartfelt expressions such as this. On another occasion, when a choir we had performing all stood up to sing their first song, Malcolm exclaimed, 'Look! The floor stood up!'

A few months into my role as Resident Musician in the aforementioned care home, I managed to persuade a famous Welsh folksinger, who was semi-retired and lived locally, to come over to entertain the residents on the last Monday afternoon of every month. While offering a varied program of events for the residents was a good thing, it was nevertheless also helpful to balance this with more regular fixtures. The Welsh folksinger was one of the more regular dates in the diary. Many of the residents at the home were Welsh speakers and were already familiar with his songs. They enjoyed singing along. These informal concerts were very popular not only amongst the residents but also amongst many nurses and carers.

The folksinger had a very relaxed and engaging demeanour and he would happily chat to the residents before and after the concert. Many would remember him from one visit to the next. It was always difficult to predict what might come out during these conversations, however. After one performance, a gentleman resident who would often wait around to have a little chat with the folk singer at the end of the concert exclaimed all of a sudden, 'My goodness – you do have *very big ears*, don't you?' The singer laughed and responded by saying, 'Do I? No one has ever mentioned that before!' At another performance, a lady had taken a fancy to him, remarking in-between the songs, 'You're a very good-looking man, aren't you?' Soon enough I'd become accustomed to such comments, but sometimes they could still take me by surprise.

While it can often be refreshing to be with people where all the rules relating to good manners and etiquette imposed by society simply don't matter anymore, who will often say exactly what comes to mind, the situation can also be quite toe-curling! Not only would high-quality performances take place in the care home. Occasionally, I would arrange to take a few of the residents with me to the nearby Arts Centre's theatre if a suitable concert was being programmed there. A short trip from the care home to the theatre would offer a welcome change to residents who were still in the early stages of dementia, providing them with a taste of 'normal' living once more.

One evening, I took Diana to see a concert by two singers from Welsh National Opera. She'd dressed up for the occasion, put on some makeup and her best jewellery. She was one of the first members of the audience to get up on her feet at the end of the concert for the standing ovation, clapping her hands animatedly. As we were leaving the theatre at the end of the concert, she turned to me and said, 'I've had a grand time.' She commented all the way home how much she had enjoyed the evening.

When I visited her the next morning after breakfast, it became clear to me that Diana remembered nothing about the previous evening's concert. I took out my mobile phone and showed a photo that I'd taken of a beaming Diana flanked by the two wonderful opera singers. She exclaimed, 'Well my god! I remember now! What a wonderful concert that was!' I printed up the photo, wrote the date and the occasion on the back, and put it up on her bedroom wall.

9. Headphones

Some families will visit with increasing rarity – a kind of prolonged cooling-off period – until they're hardly seen at all around the home. Others, however, will remain fiercely loyal to a mother or father, husband or wife, despite the harrowing and depressing fact that the disease is slowly stripping their loved ones of his or her identity and personhood in front of their very eyes.

One such relative was a sister who travelled far to visit her brother Conrad every week. Then, inexplicably, the visits suddenly stopped. When I asked after her with one of the carers, I was told that she had finally given up on Conrad. She felt she had finally lost him. The dementia had taken everything. Her brother no longer recognised her, not even briefly. It had finally reached the stage where she simply could not face visiting him. She was grieving for this loving, intelligent man that she had grown up with was now lost to her and the world around him.

Conrad had early onset Alzheimer's. He used to wonder endlessly around the care home's corridors. His focus was disarmingly short. It was as if his perception of the world was atomised into tiny fragments – briefly surfacing before being swallowed once more into the dark void of non-recognition. Engagement was very difficult. He talked, but had aphasia, which meant that most of the time the words and sentences that came out made little sense. Sometimes a shaft of intelligible light would appear from behind the clouds of forgetfulness. On one occasion, during a short one-to-one session, out of the blue, and quite clearly to my surprise, Conrad said: 'One day, I'll be back.'

Those brief moments of lucidity became rarer and rarer, however. Conrad could not stay more than a few minutes in any kind of music session. He did not respond well to one-to-one sessions either. Sometimes simply the sound of the harp playing would gently sooth some residents, but this did not seem to have much of an effect on Conrad. As time went by, his condition deteriorated. The deterioration in people with early onset Alzheimer's often seems quicker, the effect more visibly catastrophic.

In a few more months, Conrad could no longer walk unaided. His body as well as his mind was gradually locking up. His hands remained tightly shut, nails permanently digging into raw skin. His knees became permanently bent. He could not talk or walk and had to be helped with all his meals. Even basic processes such as eating became increasingly difficult.

Conrad's sister was desperate for him to receive some kind of enrichment – some respite from the dementia that was torturing him – but I just couldn't seem to get a foothold on him. I couldn't connect with Conrad. I knew that music could offer much-needed sustenance, but the music just wasn't getting through to him. The avenue of communication remained blocked. I thought I had tried everything.

But then, I had an idea. I needed to bring the music even closer to Conrad, and the only way to do this was through headphones. If this didn't work, then Conrad would be lost to music. And lost to the world.

I'd asked Conrad's sister about his musical likes and dislikes and searched for some of them on my iPad – music he used to enjoy listening to in his twenties and thirties during the 1970s and 1980s. The day had finally arrived for the two of us try out our headphones experiment with Conrad. I first checked the levels through the headphones on my own ears so that the music wasn't either too loud or too quiet. I gently placed the headphones around his ears, all the while letting him know what I was doing.

We waited to see a reaction. At first, there was no response. Not even a glimpse of recognition. The sinking, desperate feeling in my stomach that I often experienced when trying to conduct sessions with Conrad returned.

Then, after about a minute or so, Conrad brought his hands up to his head as if to remove the headphones from his ears. But just as he was about to do this, he paused momentarily, and a slow smile suddenly spread across his face as he listened to the music playing through the iPad.

The music had finally got through to him. Conrad shuffled a little closer to the edge of his seat as if trying to get up. But rather than getting up, he started coordinating his arms and feet to the rhythm and pulse of the track. We soon realised that what he was doing was miming the drums along to the track. He just sat at the edge of the seat, 'air drumming' along to a Genesis song! It was one of those breakthrough moments – as extraordinary as it was wonderful – which made my job, despite its daily frustrations and difficulties, such a rewarding experience.

The next day I bought a portable iPod for Conrad, creating a library of tracks for him to play, and filling it with all kinds of music that any of his friends and family knew he loved. Sadly, as the months went by, it became harder and harder to connect with Conrad. I talked to his sister, and we came up with a list of songs that came from when he was in his late teens, in the hope that by going back further in time we could re-establish the connections.

But Conrad no longer tried to move to the music as he had done so powerfully that first time. However, I could still see in his eyes that he was hearing and listening to the music and deriving some comfort from the experience. There were days when this was all I'd see from Conrad. Then there would be better days when a slow smile would cross his face a fleeting acknowledgement that what he was hearing was familiar to him, and that it felt good.

Conrad's sister did eventually start returning on a more regular basis. She had come to accept that things would never be as they were. Her brother would remain a mere shadow of his former self. But she had now reached some kind of acceptance and had willingly entered into this difficult, final chapter of their lives together. Music had somehow facilitated that process of acceptance, providing a crumb of certainty in an otherwise difficult and uncertain situation.

Headphones can work when all else seems to fail. This is especially the case in the later stages of dementia, when residents become either too unsettled to attend a music session or are unable to attend because they are physically incapable of doing so or are bed-bound. Headphones can prove effective when residents become very fretful, finding it very difficult to engage or are lost somewhere in their own world. When you think it's nearly impossible to reach them, music remains the best – and sometimes only – form of communication. Of course, it's important to tailor the music repertoire for each resident by asking the resident (if possible) and family members or friends of their loved ones' musical tastes, likes and dislikes.

Using headphones can also be an effective way of shutting out all that is happening around a PWD – the noise in the lounge from other residents, visiting families, the carers chatting, or the constant drone of the television from the residents' lounge.

*****

I was driving home from work one late afternoon. It was early autumn. The days were getting shorter and there was a carpet of leaves gathering along the side of the road. I switched on the radio and a song was playing that I had not heard for many, many years. The song took me right back to my childhood – being in the car with my parents and elder brother and reminding me of our annual holidays during Thanksgiving week. My father was a professional photographer with his own business in town. What with weddings and other events, the summer months were the busiest time of year for him. Therefore, family holidays were always taken during the week of Thanksgiving.

The smell of autumn in the air always reminds me of those holidays, happy and exciting times with my family. The song on the radio immediately triggered these memories and emotions for me. In an instant it took me right back. One can never underestimate the power of a song or a piece of music to act as a trigger, opening a gateway for memories, emotions, feelings and senses.

Music is like a sixth sense, bringing you back in touch with the sights, sounds, smells, tastes and touch of past experiences. Even for residents in the later stages of dementia – frail and unresponsive most of the time, like Conrad – a song, played through headphones, often draws a positive response.

10. Music and Movement

The benefits of singing in a group have already been discussed in this book in several places, especially how social activities such as singing can bring people in similar situations closer together in addition to boosting emotional wellbeing and relieving depression. Music and movement can also have a similar effect; and, like singing in a group, active participation can also be an effective means of expression.

As suggested by its name, the focus during the music and movement sessions shifts from singing to moving, with music again providing the foundations. The aim here is to slowly unfurl tired, stiff limbs, to loosen up a little, warm up. But most importantly, these sessions are designed to enjoy the moment.

Many residents are often immobile for a long time, so being able to move – maybe just a little, and even while still being seated – is important. While getting up to dance is possible for some of the other residents, a connection

– not only through voice but also through touch – is made. Many residents long for a human touch above and beyond the routine, daily touch that comes with physical care, such as washing, toileting, getting dressed and help with eating. A touch that comes through even just a small movement to music or through dance is something that both carer and resident can experience, celebrate, enjoy and share together.

Even though the focus of these sessions is primarily on movement, residents are also encouraged to sing along to the songs that are played. They are taught simple choreographic dance moves to certain songs and encouraged to act them out. Amongst the most popular songs have been 'Catch a Falling Star', sung by Perry Como, or the traditional American spiritual song 'He's Got the Whole World in His Hands'. Many of the residents who regularly come to the music and movement sessions remember the dance sequence to 'Catch a Falling Star'. Within a few seconds of hearing the opening of the song, residents will instantly recognise it. They will know what moves to make, and will be ready to go, as shown in the table on the next page.

Having conducted several music and movement sessions with more-or-less the same set of residents over a period of many months, it never ceased to fascinate me how they performed these dance sequences *without* any aid or prompting from me.

Lyrics	Residents' Physical Movements
'Catch a falling Star…'	Reach up with one arm to 'catch a star'
'…and put it in your pocket'	Tap the side of the hip to indicate a pocket
'Never let it fade away'	Hold out a hand and shake the index finger
'Catch a falling Star and put it in your pocket'	Repeat the first two gestures
'Save it for a rainy day'	Run the fingers in a downward motion to represent rain

So long as the song was playing, they could perform these gestures all on their own. And what's more, they could sing along to the recording and remember the words too. All I did was select the song to be played and just look on in amazement at these wonderful people who could learn, remember and perform these movements without any help from anyone.

A casual observer looking at the group following these dance routines for the first time could be forgiven for thinking they were just a group of ordinary elderly people having a jolly dance and a good time. Yet they all had dementia. They would forget. They had forgotten so much. If you had asked them to recite the words of 'Catch a Falling Star' without the music to sing along to, they probably wouldn't be able to do it. Yet, against all odds, they had learnt and remembered the simple sequence of movements for the song.

Songs which are good for leg movements include Frank Sinatra's 'Love and Marriage' (doing 'high' kicks during the instrumental part of the song), marching on the spot to old 'war' songs, such as 'It's a Long Way to Tipperary' or 'Pack all your Troubles'. Rock 'n' Roll songs are always popular, especially many of Elvis' hits, such as 'All Shook Up' and 'Hound Dog'. Others include 'See you Later Alligator' and 'Shake Rattle and Roll' by Bill Haley & His Comets.

Other fun songs used for music and movement have included Harry Belafonte singing 'The Banana Boat Song' and 'Jump in the Line'. Every time the line *'Come mister tally man tally me banana'* would come along, one of the male residents will always ask me for a banana immediately afterwards. I soon got into the habit of bringing a banana with me to the music and movement sessions!

Many of these songs help develop a wide and diverse range of possible movements, such as doing the twist, shaking hands, moving the neck and shoulders, clapping, reaching out with the arms and all the way down to movements involving feet and toes. Some lively songs can stimulate the participants to such an extent that they feel the urge to get up and dance.

One lady whom I escorted into the Music Room, upon hearing 'Summer Holiday' by Cliff Richard, suddenly changed her shuffling gait, straightened up and started walking perfectly to the beat of the music – I was now being led by her!

The residents suddenly feel much younger, more energised and reinvigorated. Their zest for life returns. They would get up on their feet, supported by carers or sometimes even by one another. They would be encouraged to express themselves freely through dance and movement. While I often felt exhausted at the end of a working day that had involved a music and movement session, the tiredness would always be accompanied by a very positive sense of wellbeing and accomplishment.

During these sessions I always tried to notice whether some residents came up with some interesting moves of their own, then try to copy them. I would then develop a sequence of moves that elaborated on their own ideas and incorporate them into a song. Many residents are arthritic or have long term injuries, therefore you'd need to know when not to push too hard and to listen and respect the residents' wishes if they prefer not to join in or engage in the session.

It's possible to gently coax a resident because sometimes all that's required is a soft nudge or nod of encouragement and they become fully involved in the session. However, never push anyone into doing something they simply don't want to do. People experience joy in different ways, and it's worth remembering that something can be enjoyed through passive participation by being a spectator and listening to the music.

Also, a resident who joins in and is fully engaged one week may not feel the same way the following week. We all have

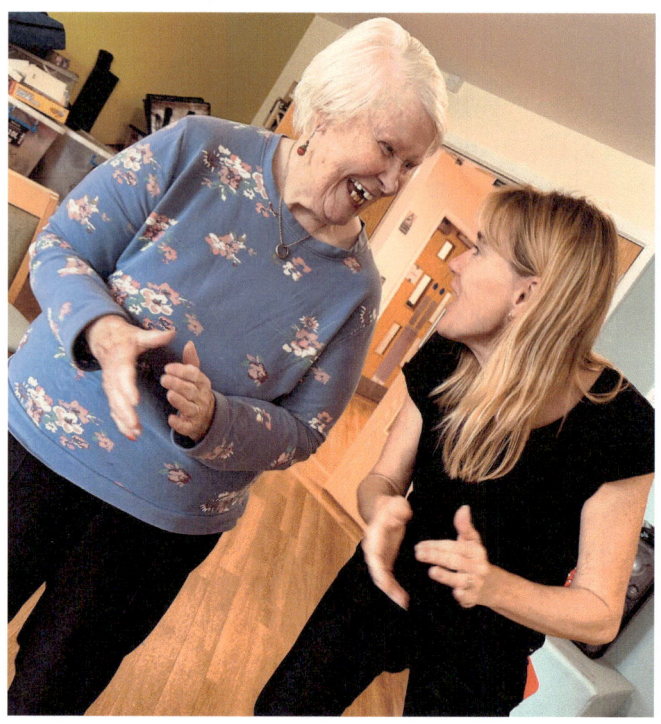

good days and bad days. Some who are perhaps initially reluctant to join in will change their minds once they see some of the other residents taking part. I would then take it gently from that point. As well as the upbeat music, traditional ballroom music is still very much enjoyed by many, and it's lovely to see residents 'in hold' – dancing the waltz – and remembering the steps, because the movement is embedded in their motor memory, which remains largely intact.[24]

---

24 This is where a specific motor task has been consolidated into the memory through frequent repetition.

A couple of care homes would pay for a dance company to come into the home every fortnight. The two dancers would play music through a loudspeaker that included anything from the Andrews Sisters to Harry Belafonte. The session would wind down towards the end with beautiful relaxing piano music by Ludovico Einaudi or Vince Hill's rendition of 'Edelweiss'. The dancers would come along to the care homes with props such as top hats, feather dusters, shimmering jingly scarfs, soft balls and a parachute-style multicoloured sheet that enabled residents to grab hold of the sides and move to the sound of the music, encouraging gentle stretching.

'I'm Forever Blowing Bubbles' was also an appropriate song to play towards the end of a session as it was quite relaxing. Plenty of bubbles would be blown during the song and most of the residents would enjoy seeing them floating around the room. Some would reach out to try to catch or burst them. I suppose it also took them back to their own childhood years ago.

There were songs we would sing unaccompanied that also included movement, such as 'Wind the Bobbin Up', 'Head, Shoulders, Knees and Toes', and the 'Hokey Dokey' – the latter also possible in a sitting position. Welsh songs such as '*Cân y Gwcw*' (The Cuckoo Song) also involved movement. These songs worked well not only for the purposes of exercising, but also to help with remembering. Hearing the music would trigger a memory of the words, which would in turn trigger a memory of the dance movement.

At the end of a music and movement session, residents would often leave the room feeling a little warmer, a little less shaky, a little less stooped, a little less stiff, a little less old, and would look altogether brighter and merrier. A sure sign of a successful session would be the number of smiles from residents leaving the music room – far more than when they were brought in at the beginning of the session.

*****

There came to the home a gentle giant of a man. Like other male members of his family, Jonny had been a professional boxer in his youth. He would love to look at old photographs of himself and other members of his family in their boxing attire. Many could be seen striking a pose wearing large, padded gloves or sporting heavy gold-and-leather belts. Jonny had a story for nearly all these photos. Looking at a photo prompted him to remember the exact names of different members of his family. He could even remember the name of the family dog. It became apparent that the stories he recited were ones he'd recited time and time again. He'd sit up in his chair and tell the story animatedly, using the same quotes, word-for-word each time.

These stories were part of Jonny's identity. Like a warm, cosy blanket, they offered him comfort, and he held on to them because they formed such an important part of his character. After all, he'd recited many of these stories throughout his lifetime. Jonny could also recite old songs from childhood, word-for-word. He also loved to sing along to a recording of Vera Lynn singing 'There'll be Blue Birds Over the White Cliffs of Dover'; although, at times, such songs would make him tearful.

Even the big, heavy boxers had to be light and nimble on their feet. Jonny often demonstrated that this element had not left him as he loved to dance. He remembered the footwork and steps to many dances, from the waltz to a quickstep to the twist and a jive. He would heave himself out of the chair with great momentum, grab the nearest female resident, help her to her feet to dance with him, and then would manoeuvre himself and his dance partner confidently around the floor.

During quieter moments, a softer and more vulnerable part of Jonny's character would come through. Dredging up those past memories would bring along an awful longing for old friends and family. Sometimes it would become just too painful for Jonny, and he would break down in tears. It became very difficult for his children to witness this when they visited regularly.

On one such occasion, to alleviate some of his distress, I took Jonny out for a stroll in the sunshine. I hoped that this might make him feel a little better. We entered the courtyard in the centre of the care home. It was awash with the early afternoon's sunshine. Standing there, the music of that morning's session came back to Jonny. We danced together to a silent soundtrack in the sunshine, the lovely music playing over and over inside his mind.

*****

When words fail, music has the power to stir, to move people to tears, to move people to dance. Music can take you back to the days you went out dancing, to concerts you used to attend, to the songs you sang your young children to sleep, or further back to your own school days, and even to the nursery rhymes sung to you by your own mother. Music stirs the emotions and stokes the memories.

Many years ago, when I'd not long realised the effect that familiar songs were having on PWD, an elderly lady was reminded of the days she used to go dancing in a village hall. On that particular occasion I had turned up to a care home to conduct a music session wearing a pair of silver ballet pumps. The elderly lady remembered walking home along a canal after the dance, carrying a pair of silver dancing shoes under her arm. The silver shoes were her pride and joy. She remembered how her boyfriend at the time snatched the shoes from her and snapped the soles before throwing them into the canal. She remembered the crack they had made when he snapped them. He was angry with her after she'd had a dance with another man. She never forgot that moment.

The combination of a certain song and the fact that I was wearing a pair of silver shoes was enough to stir her memory. She was in the later stages of dementia and conversation was very difficult. She would often ask me to sing the 'Skye Boat Song' as she said that the song reminded her of her mother and a vision she had as a child of a red coffee pot sitting proudly in the middle of the kitchen table many years ago.

11. Through a Mirror of Words

Music remains at the centre of my career as both resident and peripatetic musician, working with care homes in and around the area where I live. But while most of the music sessions I have conducted tend to focus on songs and singing, music can sometimes provide a springboard for other related activities. As seen in the last chapter on music and dance, music does not exist in isolation. Different art forms can be brought together to create new synergies, such as the 'Art in response to music' sessions set up in one of the care homes where I have worked.[25]

One of the most interesting artistic projects involved getting residents to write poems. In many ways this was a more challenging project than music because words and language are often the tools of communication that first disappear with the onset of dementia. However, I knew that words and phrases could be recovered from the mind through music. Could poetry do the same? When Welsh poet Gwion Hallam contacted me to tell me that he was

25   See Chapter 14 below.

being funded by Literature Wales to work on an eight-week community project involving poetry and dementia, I was intrigued to find out how it would all work. He was due to visit two residential homes, spending most of his time at one of the care homes where I worked.

During this period, Gwion spoke at length to some of the residents who'd agreed to be part of the project. He encouraged them to share stories about their lives, and in the case of one resident, his particular love of poetry. Gwion then set about to write a poem that was based on his experiences of engaging and collaborating with the residents. The poem, originally written in Welsh, translates as 'Through a Mirror'.[26]

Before starting work on the poem itself, Gwion worked with around eight residents individually, creating free-form poems in *vers libre* that used some of the residents' own words and expressions. Once completed, the poems were then presented to the residents. Many were placed on the residents' bedroom walls. Since many of the residents were Welsh speakers, most of Gwion's poems were written in Welsh. (There has, in fact, been a strong and important Bardic tradition in Wales that dates back to the sixth century.) Nevertheless, some poems were also written in English, including the following by Christine called 'Things to Do', which depicts the fragmented mind of a person with dementia:

---

26   The poem was adjudged to have been the best in the Crown Competition at the 2017 National Eisteddfod, held that year on Anglesey.

Things to do

Well, I've got two girls
Hong Kong and Shanghai
and writing and drawing
and going for walks

and things;

like using my son's car
and a swimming bath
and television,
yes, I like watching it.
Both my parents are Scottish
and then there is John;
he's a lovely boy
but won't be here till Friday
well, he is very busy
in the university
doing everything –
arithmetic mainly.
But he'll go to those girls
and get their door open.
Does anything open
anymore?
Arithmetic was my best subject
at Amersham Grammar School –
war time it was –
we did all sorts of things
but arithmetic gave me

more than anything
else. And English
and French and Geography too
and History and English
but cookery yes
was my favourite thing,
as well.
I'll go do some cookery
and John, he can help me
and there's a lady called Jan
with bread and things
and blankets and sheets
and jumpers and skirts
and all sort of things
and bathing suits too
I embroidered at home,
and things like this blouse –
I had a machine of it all.
(where is it?)
My home?
It's in London
and Amersham,
Chesham
and Latimer –
that's a watery place,
and Wales
is quite interesting,
John lives there a lot.
I've travelled a lot,
I like Geography most
he's a lovely boy

and he'll be here on Saturday,
always.
(you've travelled?)

To London and Amsterdam,
yes, I've been far,
in my father's car usually,
as far as Little Chalfont
and back.

Chris (February 2017)

When Christine's son, John, read the poem he became quite emotional. But at the same time, he was also amazed at just how many things his mother could remember. On the surface, the poem may have come across as a rather random and haphazard series of disconnected thoughts and impressions. In fact, it made a lot of sense to John, and he felt comforted by the fact that his mother still remembered so many things from her past. They may have become rather jumbled in her mind, but they were still there: they still formed an important part of who Chris was – and had been – as a person.

What amazed me was that each poem created during the project was testament to the residents' prevailing memories. Their thoughts and impressions, now placed down in black and white, on paper, was something solid to keep hold of when everything else appeared to be slowly slipping away.[27]

---

27 Gwion continued to visit the care home for a while, having forged strong connections with both residents and carers.

12. 'Moon River'

I was not having a good day. The last thing I felt like doing was singing. However, being in the company of residents that I'd worked with for many months, or in some cases several years, somehow lifted me. It was a levelling feeling being in their company. This was their life, or all that was left of it. They were no longer part of the world outside of those walls. My 'bad' day seemed so inconsequential here.

Most of these residents had lived lives that were – in one way or another – rich and rewarding. As doctors, teachers, nurses and lawyers, many of them had made important contributions to society. Their world had now shrunk due to a shrinking brain. There were many times when I felt lucky and privileged to be doing what I did, because often I received so much in return by giving a music session or being able to spend time with residents individually. I received their love and laughter, their hopes and fears.

More than anything else, perhaps, I received their complete trust and friendship.

There is one person who particularly comes to mind here. Let me introduce you to Raymond. Raymond was one of thousands of children evacuated from Liverpool during the Second World War. He was just four years old at the time. Many children from Liverpool were evacuated to North Wales, but Raymond and his little sister were separated during the evacuation. Both his parents were lost during the bombings. He occasionally talked about this episode in his life with me and often wondered about his sister.

Raymond had both Parkinson's disease and Korsakoff Syndrome – the latter due to many years of alcohol abuse. He could be quite unsteady on his feet, at times losing his balance and walking with a lilt.[28] In many such cases, it was almost as if the person's 'spirit level' – that part of the brain that kept himself or herself on an even keel – had been damaged.[29]

There were times when I'd see Raymond for the vast majority of a day. Not only would he attend my music session, but he'd also have a one-to-one session with me, which usually involved going for a walk. Plus, later, he'd join me for a session with some of the other residents. There were other times when I wouldn't see Raymond for

28 This could be an indication of damage to the part of the brain which is responsible for movement.

29 Oliver Sacks' 'On the Level', from *The Man Who Mistook his Wife for a Hat* (Picador Classics, 1985), pp. 67–72.

several weeks, apart from when I'd pop my head around his bedroom door to see how he was.

Sometimes Raymond took himself off to bed in a dementia-induced self-imposed exile. There he would stay, alone, for many weeks. The reason for this 'all or nothing' interaction was because of Raymond's hypomania episodes.[30] He would either be up for any music sessions and activities going that day ... or up for nothing at all.

Raymond would remember that I'd come to ask how he was, but no amount of coaxing would rouse him from his chair or bed. And yet I always sensed that he would be back when he was good and ready. I used to joke with him: 'Have you been hibernating again Ray?' He would laugh heartily, then say, 'I'm back now!'

And it was good to have him back. When he was 'up', he was impatient to get things done, to go to places. He would ask a carer to shave him and put on some clean clothes, ready for the morning session or an afternoon concert. If I said we'd go for a walk after lunch, he would be sitting ready in his coat and hat, raring to go. As we went companionably on our little walkabout around the grounds of the home, he'd smile and greet everyone eagerly as we passed.

One of the likely symptoms of Korsakoff syndrome are fluctuating extremes in personality. On the one hand, a person may become totally disinterested in everything;

---

30   Episodes of elevated mood, being talkative, possibly decreasing when in need of sleep.

but on the other, the same person may then suddenly seem interested in absolutely everything – asking so many questions and being incredibly talkative.

One of Raymond's most favourite songs to sing was 'Moon River'. He could remember every single word to this song, although he would sometimes worry that he'd forgotten them. Then, once he'd start singing, all the words would come flooding back. He would often sing this song during a music session. And if there was a concert in the home and Raymond was up and about, he would happily stand up and perform his rendition of 'Moon River' in front of the other residents. A wonderful smile would spread across his face as everyone would applaud at the end. He was the star of the show, and he loved it!

I noticed that when I once gave him a microphone to sing into, Raymond seemed much steadier while holding it. His tremors became less obvious. It was as if the task of doing something that he enjoyed – like singing – which took his whole focus, seemed to relax him, and his tremors subsided.

One day, when we were on our way out to the garden and in the lift taking us down to the ground floor, Raymond caught sight of himself in the mirror in the lift and exclaimed, 'Bloody hell, is that me nurse?' (He would always call me nurse, even though I explained to him many times that I wasn't one!) He paused, then said: 'Good God, I look a bloody fright!' I couldn't help myself but to start laughing at this comment. He started to laugh along too. 'Come along,' I said, 'Let's enjoy ourselves this afternoon while we can!'

Raymond was aware that his drinking had made him the way he was. The loss of weight. The forgetfulness. The personality swings. It partly explained the minimal contact he received from his son. There would be weeks when he would withdraw into his room, until the point where I'd almost lose hope of encountering the Raymond of old. Then one day I would come to work to find a note on my desk from one of the carers, which said, 'Can you please print some lyric sheets of Ray's favourite songs please'. And with that note, I knew that he was back, at least for the time being.

Amongst the barrage of questions and phrases that I'd receive from Raymond on a daily basis were the following ones:

'What's wrong with me?'
'How old am I?'
'Do you drink … I used to drink a lot.'
'Where's my son? Why does he never come to see me?'
'Am I married? Is my wife dead … I think she is, you know.'
'It's terrible not being able to remember.'
'Why am I here?'
'How old are you? Forty-nine? Me too! We're the same age!'
'Do you have a car? Did you drive to work? Can we go for a drive in your car?'

'Do I still have my house? Who's living in my house now?' And so it went on …

There was a day during summer when we were sitting outside in the sunshine, I'd lent him my sunglasses and he wore a straw hat on his head to protect himself from the sun. Both of us had rolled up our trousers to hopefully get a little suntan on our legs. A carer took a photo of us sitting side-by-side like this, and Raymond had this photo up in his room for several years.

The usual questions were asked again.

Then, after a while, he leaned forward, hands folded together on his legs. He remained quiet for a while. He seemed lost in thought. Then, looking down at the ground, he said quietly under his breath, 'I was cruel, you know.' I wasn't sure whether he was directing the comment at me or just saying it to himself. He was referring to his family, but he didn't go on, and neither did I pursue this line of conversation. I could speculate to myself that this may have been the reason why his son rarely visited, even though he didn't live very far away. What he disclosed to me at that moment probably related to the alcohol abuse that had affected his family at the time. Saddest of all, he also seemed to be reflecting that maybe it wasn't too late to make things better.

As already mentioned, there were times when I didn't see Raymond for many weeks. He would be 'hibernating', as he and I would call it. But it still saddened me that here was this man who clearly saw me as his close friend yet would just as soon disappear into a dark chasm where it was impossible to reach him.

Until, without warning or prompting, he would suddenly reappear again – talkative, funny, humorous, asking those endless questions. Unique and unforgettable. My friend, Raymond …

13. Nursing the Nurses

As you might expect, there are always going to be nurses present in a nursing home. However, what you might not have expected was that most of these nurses made up a significant percentage of the residents in one of the care homes I worked. These were of course retired nurses who had, in the course of time, succumbed to dementia. It was always sobering and poignant to see so many people in the healthcare profession who had been involved in that line of work for many years, caring for others. Now they themselves were being cared for in nursing or care homes.

Was it their condition that had brought them here, together? Of these nurses, I found out through family members that almost all of them had worked night shifts on a regular basis during their careers as nurses. I mentioned at the start of this book that I was going to leave the science to the scientists. However, in the work that I do, after a while, some things simply scream out at you. You just can't help noticing a certain trend or pattern. I am convinced that there must be some kind of link between the stressful careers of nurses – especially those who have often worked night shifts – and the onset of dementia later in life. It can't just simply be a coincidence. The figures would surely be too high.

Needing further proof than simply relying on what I'd observed empirically in one or two homes, I took time to call other care homes to ask about residents' past professions before illness or retirement. As expected, many of their residents used to be nurses. Furthermore, many of them used to be nurses who regularly worked night shifts.

Numerous research has emphasised the importance of a good night's sleep. Ideally, this should be between seven and nine hours of good quality, undisturbed sleep per night. At Rochester University, New York, Maiken Nedergaard and a team of researchers conducted a range of experiments on people's sleep patterns. What came out of the research was that a good night's sleep acted as a kind of 'dishwasher' for the brain, helping to clean the brain of amalgamates and plaques, which is the main cause of various forms of dementia.[31]

What I often find is that the caring side of some of the retired nurses shines through in their own illness. Having spent years in the profession, this side of their character doesn't just disappear. They have spent many years caring in this way and now they are being cared

31   Makine Nedergaard, 'Garbage Truck of the Brain', *Science* (28 June 2013), vol. 340/6140, pp. 1529–1530.

for themselves in the nursing home. One case where the caring side was still very present in her character was Daisy.[32] She would patiently assist residents with their meals, guide others along the hallways, or help a person in need of assistance to walk to a chair and ensure they were sitting down comfortably. She would push other residents in a wheelchair, comfort residents who were restless, frightened or vexed, and all this even though she was suffering and was damaged too.

In truth, Daisy had never forgotten she was a nurse, but there had been a history of mental illness and depression in her life going back many years. It became apparent to her son that the mental illness was kept under control to an extent, mainly by the love and support of Daisy's husband. However, when Daisy's husband passed away quite suddenly some years previously, things started to unravel in her life. Daisy had, in essence, lost her soulmate, her guardian and her anchor. She became desperately lost and lonely and became increasingly dependent on her only son.

As her only child, Daisy's son, in turn, had found caring for her enormously stressful. It was clear to him that Daisy desperately longed for her lost husband. She could not cope without her son constantly by her side and her demands gradually became too much for him. By conducting a little research, her son subsequently found out that his mother had suffered from mental illness since her late teens.

---

32 Daisy is also mentioned in Chapter 18.

She was extremely close to her husband, and her son therefore came to the conclusion that he had protected her, had kept her generally happy and content so that she functioned from day to day and held a job which she'd enjoyed for many years as a district nurse. Her husband had nursed the nurse throughout her life and career; but once he was gone there was no-one else there to protect Daisy.

She would often tell me how she had travelled around and met many people in the area due to her profession. She once said, 'People were kind to me, you know. So very kind.' I believe Daisy thrived on the kindness she received. It was important for her own wellbeing and fuelled her thirst for life. She received it from her husband and longed for it from her son.

It was more than he could deliver in the end. Daisy craved attention and kindness in the care home and could recognise this longing in others. It explained why she continued to care for other residents even when she had become a resident herself.

14. Art in Response to Music[33]

There were occasions when I would work in a care home with a local artist. Painting is an activity that many people with dementia can partake in, experiencing enjoyment in the process. This is discussed briefly in Joseph Jebelli's book *In Pursuit of Memory: The Fight Against Alzheimer's*, where he states that, 'Painting stimulates the parietal lobe, a region involved in creativity and one that remains intact until quite late in the disease.'[34]

During these art sessions, we would occasionally combine it with music, calling them 'Art in Response to Music'. These sessions entailed small groups of residents sitting around a table with paper, pencils, chalk, paint, brushes, and water to clean the brushes. I would sit nearby, either playing the harp or piano, improvising most of the time and usually not singing. The music was designed to provide a relaxing backdrop to the residents' artistic endeavours with brush, paint and canvas.

33   This chapter is based on an article I wrote for *The Journal of Dementia Care,* March/April 2021 Vol. 29, No. 2.
34   Joseph Jebelli, *In Pursuit of Memory: The Fight Against Alzheimer's* (John Murray, 2017), p. 101.

Usually, the artist who had come in for the session took a very laid back approach, retiring into the background and letting the residents paint only if they wished. Light encouragement was provided only when needed. Sessions using modelling clay also proved to be effective, with the participating residents creating little bowls or quirky figures. Some preferred to colour-in with special adult colouring books while others seemed to enjoy trying to copy another picture or to paint a still-life, such as a vase of flowers.

Some seemed as if they were afraid to paint or draw on blank canvas, unsure of what they would produce, feeling unable to, or being conscious of not being able to produce a decent piece of art.

However, the most interesting work was created by those residents who would paint onto completely blank paper while I played some music in the background. The results of these sessions were both varied and often fascinating pieces of abstract art, and arguably provided some revealing insights into those residents' minds.

Some would combine their drawings with writings. Garbled thoughts and messages were transferred onto paper in a creative form that combined words and letters with shapes and colours. Some would use paint to create a wash of different colours with no discernible shape or form. A few residents would regularly join the session but preferred not to partake in any painting. Some were physically incapable of doing so. Instead, they seemed to enjoy listening to the music and watching the other residents participate in an often relaxed atmosphere.

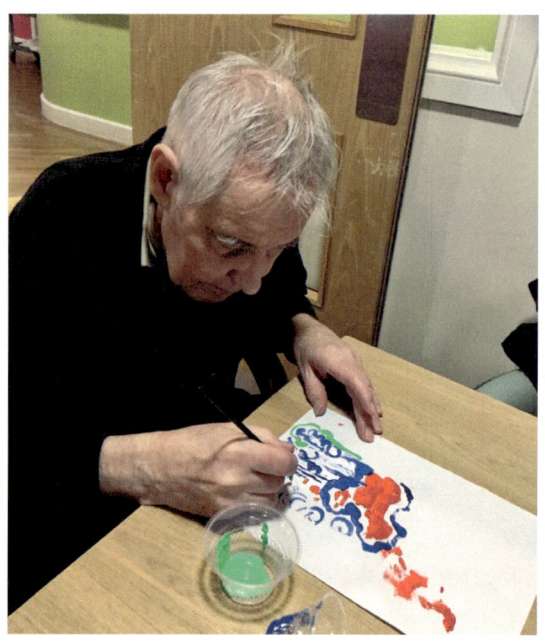

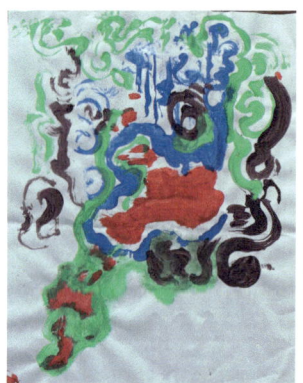

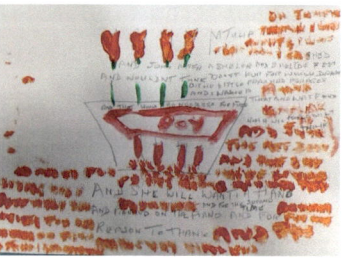

Myrtle, who preferred to use blank paper during these sessions, possessed a very distinct style. Her paintings usually comprised many individual little drawings dotted around the same piece of paper. There was something very 'detached' about her style. Some of the images looked a little like insects or flowers. Others took on the character of symbols of various sorts. Most of them were painted in different colours, with a surprising level of detail in many cases.

I found out that Myrtle worked as a clerk in the military for over twenty years. Her training had taken her to such far-away places as Indonesia and Singapore. I wondered whether these drawings were somehow linked to her military past? It was difficult to say. I noticed quite soon after meeting Myrtle that she did not like to see herself in the mirror. Neither did she seem to like to see herself in a photograph that might have been taken during one of the art sessions. When she walked past a mirror, her smile would suddenly fade, and it would be replaced suddenly by a scowl.

The reason for this was not known. It could be that Myrtle simply did not like to see herself aged – or did not recognise herself – even though she looked physically well. She would often move things about the place. I'd come into work one day to find someone's family photographs on my desk. Next to it would be a half-eaten biscuit, an odd sock or a slipper.

My work diary – which that had gone missing for many weeks, to the point where I'd finally given up on seeing it ever again and had bought a new one – was suddenly back! It would then be a case of spending the next half hour trying to solve the mystery of whose family the photographs belonged to, who was missing a pink sock or a blue fluffy slipper, or cracking the mystery behind the strange return of my long-lost diary.

All of this was grist to Myrtle's amusement. She loved animals and enjoyed the voluntary dog visits to the care home very much. She would often be seen walking around the corridors with a stuffed animal tucked under her arm, talking and smiling to it. Her room was an Aladdin's cave of stuffed animals. Many were probably gathered from other residents' rooms! I often brought my own little French bulldog into work and Myrtle adored him. She would clasp her hands in delight when she saw him. She seemed to recognise him straightaway. If I had not brought him into work for a while, she would turn to me and ask, 'Where's the little black dog?'

*****

One morning, Jimmy was brought up to the music room to try his hand at an 'Art in Response to Music' session. He was never too fussed about music sessions, singing along to 'Molly Malone' and 'My Bonny Lies Over the Ocean' if the mood happened to take him. At first, he was reluctant to participate in the art session, commenting, 'I'm not a child you know!' However, after a short while, he decided to paint a little and seemed to be enjoying himself. Jimmy started relaxing into the music I was playing on the piano while continuing to paint.

Then he started talking and reminiscing about the Second World War. This was a topic that Jimmy usually avoided talking about and the carers respected this. It wasn't a subject that we would normally raise with him. However, during this particular session, he started to tell me a little about his life during the war. He told me he was a gunner in the RAF. The more Jimmy talked, the more obvious it became that he had been deeply affected by this particular period in his life. He reflected, 'It makes me sad to think how many people I must have killed. They had families too. I worry that I might have killed some of my own.' He sighed before saying, 'You know, I was only a baby myself. I was just a teenager.'

Jimmy went on to say that he had spent time in prison camps in France, Belgium and Germany for many years during the war. The session had somehow prompted Jimmy to open up about his past. He had revisited memories that were both painful and difficult to forget. 'I had twelve brothers and sisters', he reflected. 'Some of them died in the war, but I don't like to talk about that. It makes me too sad.' Then he paused again, before looking directly at me and saying. 'I don't believe in God, you know. How could God let something like that happen, and keep happening?'

15. Bridging the Generations

The little boy had spotted Annie sitting by the table and immediately ran over to her. He swiftly climbed up onto her knee. She welcomed him with open arms and anointed him on the top of his head with a gentle kiss. Annie was not the little boy's grandmother or his great aunt. In fact, they were not related at all. This was only the third time they'd ever met, but they'd bonded while working on a craft and music project in the care home.

Annie's bond with the little boy was not an isolated experience. Young children and residents would experience complete and unencumbered joy in each other's company while working on an art collage or while singing songs together. We'd often invite local children from preschool years to come in. Primary and secondary schools would often visit care homes to give a short concert or to work together on a project with residents over several weeks that would often involve arts and crafts, and/or music.

At national and local level, through government white papers and local council policies, the benefits of developing relationships between young children and the elderly under one roof is finally being grasped and valued. More and more day care and residential care homes for the elderly are incorporating inter-generational interaction as part of their care plans. There are examples of kindergartens opening up in care homes in the USA and Canada, with numerous clips appearing on YouTube showing the effectiveness and benefits of this concept.

The benefits could also extend very effectively to PWD. When I first mooted the possibility of bringing in children to interact with residents who had dementia, some were naturally concerned about how they would react to people with short-term memory loss, who appeared confused and often talked in a language that made no sense. How might a child respond to an elderly person being seen wandering about the place? What might happen if something was said that might offend a child?

Clearly the whole process had to be carefully monitored and observed. However, under the watchful eye of carers both for the children and the residents, this coming together of PWD and children was a positive and very rewarding experience for all involved. There are so many people living with dementia in society today. It is therefore likely that children will have encountered relatives who have some form of dementia. Spending time on a regular basis with PWD can help remove any stigma that children may have developed towards dementia.

Of course, the whole process is more carefully managed than simply filling a room full of children and residents then sitting back and seeing what might transpire. Even before the children are allowed to meet the residents, they are given a little talk about dementia, so they have some idea what to expect. For example, they are told not to be surprised if they are called by another name as there is always a chance that a resident may recognise them as someone else. Children are reminded that it's not unusual for a resident to ask the same question repeatedly, or for a resident to use words they may not understand.

During the initial first meeting both the children and residents approach the situation cautiously. Both sides are unsure what to expect. Some residents are reluctant to become involved and simply aren't that keen to mix with children. But then something quite special happens which is difficult to put into words. I have seen it taking shape before my very eyes during those first meetings. A connection is formed. It seems to me that there lies a natural affinity between a young child and a person with dementia. Even children and residents who initially show little interest in coming together seem to draw each other out. In each other's company they seem to relax and start to enjoy the experience.

How does this happen? What seems to bring the old and the young together in this way? It can be argued that PWD are also children, to some extent. They no longer behave in the way society demands from (or expects of) them. Likewise, young children are coming to terms with the rules and regulations that society dictates, the do's and don'ts, if you like. Children grow up constantly having to readjust to expected patterns of behaviour. In both the young and the old there is no pretence, no facade: a sincere and honest meeting between vulnerable people, albeit generations apart.

The yawning generation gap notwithstanding, they will both say what is on their minds, and one sees and hears the 'freedom' of interaction and communication that takes place in these special gatherings. Within minutes, both generations are chatting away. Little children climb up on the residents' knees to the residents' utter delight.

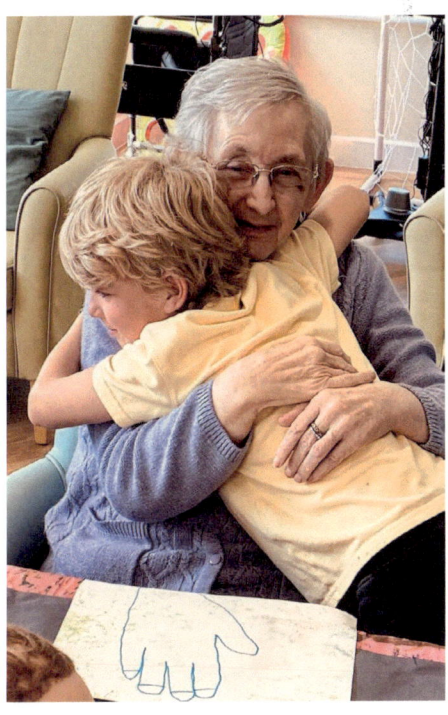

The old suddenly feel a little bit younger again, and the warm blush of youth returns momentarily to their faces. You only need to look around to see the enjoyment experienced by all participants. In most cases, residents adore seeing the children arrive and then spending time getting to know them. From my observation, it is an extremely positive experience to bring children into the homes of PWD.

To conclude this chapter, here is an example of the unique bond formed by the interaction between young and old. A short project was run by a theatre company and myself involving some of the residents and their grandchildren (and even great-grandchildren in some cases), getting them to work together over two separate Saturday sessions by creating puppets. The daughter of one of the participating residents noted that her ten-year-old daughter would get very upset when visiting her grandmother in the care home. She said that her daughter found it very difficult to get used to the fact that her grandmother had dementia and seeing her become confused and forgetful.

Through working on the project together over a couple of weeks, it succeeded in bringing the granddaughter closer to her beloved grandmother once more, and to see that she continued to be capable of living her life despite her dementia. Following the project, the granddaughter would no longer get upset when visiting her grandmother at the care home.

16. The Jazz Man and the Trumpet Man

These days, many dementia care homes have 'memory boxes'. Fitted with a Perspex window, the small wooden boxes are attached outside each resident's room, next to the door. Each box is unique and personalised to reflect the life of the occupant. Most memory boxes contain photographs, personal trinkets and mementos, testimony to a full and rich life the person would have lived before dementia gradually and cruelly put a halt to her or his 'normal' living.

There are photographs of people getting married, holidays taken with young children, the family at home celebrating Christmas, a family pet playing in the garden, a picnic in the countryside or a trip to the seaside. Many of the photographs are faded and yellowed with time, corners curling up, forming little patterns in the rich tapestry of a life well-lived. And there are photographs of the residents when they were older, too, quite possibly oblivious to the dementia that loomed, threatening their lives and dashing any hopes of a happy retirement with loved ones.

In one particular box, in one particular home, there was a black and white photograph of a handsome man in his thirties with beautiful wavy black hair slicked back fashionably. He was blowing into a clarinet, eyes squeezed closed, unperturbed that he was being photographed. He was lost in the moment and in the music.

This was Clive, a gentleman in the truest sense of the word. Softly spoken, quiet and polite, he would use his hands a great deal when trying to explain things. I knew him over several years, from when he first arrived at the care home – being able to walk and talk – to when he succumbed to the later stages of dementia, catheterised, unable to walk and weighing half the weight he was when he first came into the home.

It had always been rather difficult to hold a conversation with Clive. He fumbled with words and sometimes hallucinated, making communication challenging. His vascular dementia caused him to have an impaired ability of speech, what is often referred to as 'aphasia': he lived in poverty of vocabulary. He also suffered from apraxia, where typically he'd be unable to perform tasks or movements when asked. Both aphasia and apraxia are often associated with various forms of dementia due to the damage it causes to certain parts of the brain.

As the photo showed, Clive used to play clarinet in a jazz band, and although he would not be able to talk about it very well due to the effects of aphasia and memory loss, he did enjoy attending the music sessions. He would often sing along to the songs he knew, and I noticed that he would often harmonise the main melody too. I learnt that Clive also spoke German and Irish Gaelic. I discovered this during the music sessions. Whilst singing a popular Irish song, suddenly Clive's face would light up and he'd start speaking in Irish Gaelic! Seeing me looking at him in utter astonishment and bewilderment, he'd then throw me a mischievous wink!

Considering his aphasia, this was quite astonishing. A familiar song enabled him to tap into hidden reserves of memory that had ceased functioning in non-musical contexts and situations. Sometime later, during another session, Clive surprised me, this time by turning to German. It sounded quite fluent to me!

Even though Clive came from a musical background his apraxia resulted in coordination problems. This meant that he found it difficult to know what to do with a simple percussion instrument such as a tambourine and had to be shown how to use it. During one particular music session, I gave Clive a harmonica to try to play, but rather than hold it horizontally as one might usually do, and blow into it, he held it vertically and tried to bite into it. Maybe he was getting it confused with a clarinet, which is also held lengthways rather than widthways.

One morning I popped my head around the door of Clive's lounge. He was now in the later stages of his dementia and had been particularly unwell for many days. I noticed that a loud and unfriendly chat show was being shown on the TV in the corner. I walked over and switched it immediately to one of the classical music radio channels. The final movement of Mozart's Horn Concerto was in full flow, and as I walked out, I could hear Clive starting to sing along to the familiar melody with his face turned towards the radio. I rarely saw him in the large group music sessions towards the end of his life, but he still responded to smaller sessions in the lounge, or to one-to-ones, and continued to enjoy and appreciate good music.

*****

Mathew was in the much earlier stages of dementia. In his words, he was a 'semi-professional trumpet player' and used to play in a successful dance band. He was one of few residents who would actually state every so often that he had dementia. He was conscious that his memory was failing him. But since he was only in the earlier stages of dementia, we could still have some interesting conversations about his musical passion for trumpets and trumpeters.

He'd become very animated when talking about his trumpet-playing idols, famous players such as Harry James and Derek Watkins. We would then watch endless clips of them playing on YouTube, and he'd be delighted not only because he could listen to all his all-time favourites, but also, in most cases, he could actually see them play too! He could name the piece being played in a split second, along with its composer – faster than most contestants would have been able to do in the music round on BBC2's *University Challenge*!

He taught me to listen out for the high notes being played, loud and clear, he taught me to identify the many techniques used by the trumpeter, such as double-tonguing. He loved listening and watching Harry James' brilliant rendition of Rimsky Korsakov's 'Flight of the Bumblebee'. Mathew would sit in awe at the extraordinary feat of virtuosic technique and musicianship, iPad on his lap, watching and listening intensely as Harry James raced through the piece at a blistering pace. The delight that lit up his face made my day, and I looked forward to each and every session with Mathew. It was inspirational to see people like him respond to music in this way.

I knew of a gifted young trumpet player called Owain who lived in a village not far from the care home where Mathew resided. Owain had successfully competed in several regional and national music competitions and was planning on auditioning for a place in one of the country's top music conservatoires. I decided to get in touch with Owain to ask him whether he'd be interested in coming to meet Mathew, and of course to bring his trumpet with him. Owain agreed to come along and meet Mathew, and so a date and time was set.

Mathew looked forward in anticipation of Owain's visit for several days. It was a cold, blustery and wet Sunday afternoon in late November. Autumnal leaves carpeted the grounds outside the care home, and the evening's darkness was already visible, threatening the grey skies in the mid-afternoon's half-light. When I arrived at the home, I was surprised to see that Owain had already arrived with his grandfather and was seated, deep in conversation with Mathew, the trumpet still lying in its case between them.

As I walked into the little lounge, Mathew immediately announced with a twinkle in his eye, 'He's here!' They had been discussing their favourite trumpet players and continued to do so until Owain offered to bring out the trumpet. Mathew sat at the edge of his seat while watching Owain blow quietly and steadily into the trumpet to warm up the instrument. He then proceeded to play several pieces for Mathew, each followed by a joint dissection and appraisal of the music by both. It was like being in a music masterclass!

Mathew marvelled at the young trumpet player's ability, technique and tone, and the joy of the afternoon's entertainment could be seen clearly on his face. When the time came to pack up the trumpet, he turned to me, whispering beneath his breath, 'He's a far better trumpeter than I ever was! He could definitely be a professional ...' Mathew referred to Owain as his 'friend' when he said he hoped the young player might visit him again. And, indeed, Owain visited Mathew several times; so he too, had also made a new friend.

What I found heartening from Owain's visit was that it showed so wonderfully the contribution that PWD can continue to give people from other walks of life. It's important that we realise PWD still have much to offer. Sharing their experiences with other people while it's still possible for them to do so is such a precious gift, especially when those experiences are shared with the younger generation. Both sides can learn from each other.

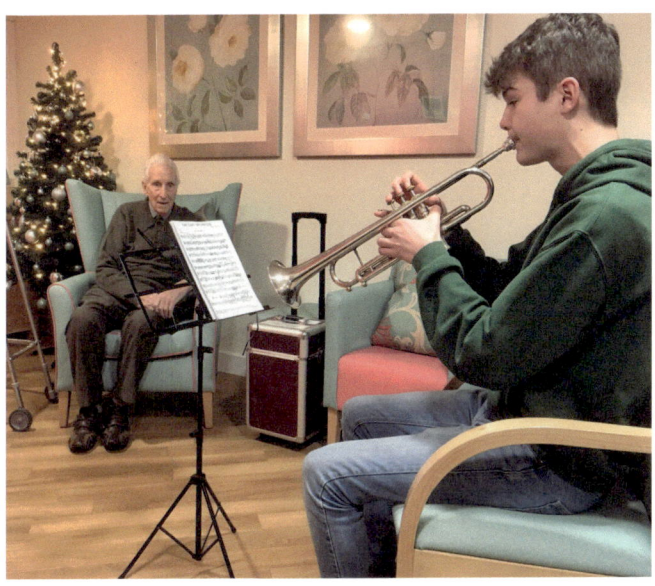

Mathew seemed totally aware that he had dementia and conceded to the fact that he would often forget things. He would shrug it off by explaining, 'It's this dementia, you know. It's a real nuisance.' But inevitably there were times when he seemed unaware that he was muddled. Once Mathew talked about a classic car he had owned, stating that he'd given the car to his son many, many years previously, and that it had probably been sold by now. However, the very next day, he said that the car was probably still in his garage, and that his son – whom he thought was in his late teens – was a little too young to be driving such a powerful car! Time seemed to have eluded and deluded him – his son had snowy white hair and had retired several years ago.

17. 'Run Rabbit Run!'

There isn't much of a connection to music in this short chapter about Phillis, but she was one of those residents who stood out for me, perhaps because of a shared interest that wasn't, in this case, to do with music.

Phillis arrived at the nursing home wearing a pair of jeans, sweatshirt and a pair of trainers on her feet. But she wasn't in her thirties or forties. Phillis was in her mid-nineties. However, she looked not a day older than seventy-five. She used to run marathons and even skied until a year before arriving at the care home. She did not take up running seriously until she was well into her sixties. However, she broke many records in her late running career because of her age.

While Phillis's body had remained lean, fit and healthy, her mind had become scrambled and lost. Dementia can truly be the cruellest of all diseases. Phillis's body would never again experience the freedom it once had, because her mind had become her prison.

Since Phillis was used to being very much 'on the go', she did not settle at all well in the nursing home. She could not be coaxed into attending any of the music sessions. She would remain restless and agitated most of the day. Since she had loved the outdoors so passionately, I presumed that she would come outside with me for walks around the grounds. However, she refused any invitation to go outside.

Why was it so difficult to persuade her to come outside? Her restless, confused mind would not allow her to think that this could be a positive experience and a good pastime for her to enjoy.

Then, one particular afternoon, with some gentle coaxing on my behalf, I managed to bring Phillis down to the lobby of the nursing home. She would not have gone through the final set of doors had they not happened to be automatic ones which opened as soon as we stood directly before them.

A wash of cool wind and instant warmth of the early spring sun fell on Phillis's face, immediately transforming her to a calmer more contented state. We stepped outside and finally took a walk. Soon enough she started chatting to me, listening when I told her about my own running interests. At last, she was somewhere where she felt at home – and that was being outdoors. Having spent a long while outside, walking and chatting, she returned indoors with me quite happily.

Apart for the obvious health benefits, running gives people a feeling of freedom and achievement. No matter what I've done during the day, or how busy I've been, if I manage to fit a run into my day, then – for me – it's the most important thing. Because, without a healthy mind and body, I can't function normally. Running, they say, is good for a healthy body and mind, which, in Phillis's case may seem a little ironic – maybe the seeds of Alzheimer's were already planted in Phillis's brain even before she started running in her sixties; but, who knows, it's possible that the disease was kept at bay for longer because of her active lifestyle.

Both the carers, myself and her elderly husband often tried in vain to take Phillis outside, knowing how much she would enjoy the experience once we'd reach the automatic doors, and they'd open up before her. However, Phillis became increasingly fretful, and the task of getting her outside became increasingly harder.

It was during one of her many walks around the corridors of the care home that Phillis fell and broke her hip. She was taken to hospital, and when she returned a couple of weeks later, Phillis became bed-bound. It worried me to see Phillis unable to move from the bed, as here was a woman who was used to being on her feet. Her saving grace, if one could call it that, was that she could still walk.

However, when the capacity to walk was taken away from her too, she went downhill quickly. The pain of seeing her stuck in bed was etched on her husband's face during his visits, and it was heart-breaking to see his response. I wish I could say that she got better, but there was nothing that could be done, and Phillis passed away just a few weeks after her fall.

Of course, words of comfort such as 'it was a blessing that she did not suffer too much in the end', or 'it was a good thing that Phillis was not bedridden for months' were brought out after she died. But nothing can take away the fact that dementia, in all its various diseases, is a cruel, ravaging disease. Like any disease, it cares not what kind of human being it affects, or of the devastating destruction it finally subjects to both mind and body.

18. 'Driving Miss Daisy'

One sunny afternoon, I took a resident for a spin in my car. I'd promised to take her once the weather had improved. Daisy remembered my promise and so it was arranged. However, when the day came and Daisy was safely ensconced next to me in the passenger's seat, all she did from the outset was to complain that her eyesight was poor, and she could not see the lovely landmarks along where the drive was taking her.

My so called 'good deed of the day' felt a bit flat, especially when she said at the end, 'I don't know why you bothered to take me out in the car if you weren't going to take me home!' Daisy seemed more miserable than before we set off. I suppose I don't always get things right all the time, despite my best intentions!

I suppose that going for a spin in the car was my idea of giving the residents a break from the care home and its other residents. Of course, this is not always possible due to the physical side of things, and even despite the best of my intentions, it doesn't always work out as expected. However, it's definitely worth a try, especially when I can play some of their favourite music along the way to sing along to.

There was a resident who was staying in a care home while recovering from a particularly nasty fall down the stairs of her home. She'd broken many bones, lost many teeth, and had hit her head badly during the fall. After many months recovering in the hospital, Eileen, who was in her sixties, was advised to recover somewhere for a period of convalescence before returning to her home.

To this day, I can't understand why her daughter had decided that a private nursing home was the best place for her convalescing mother, which mainly catered for elderly people with mid- to late-stage dementia. I suppose the modern care home seemed an attractive, nice place at first. But here was a woman who could still use her mobile phone, who could read novels, who yearned for a decent conversation, and felt that – apart from the carers – there was nobody there that she could talk to who made very much sense.

Granted, she was a little unsteady on her feet and a little forgetful and fretful, but this home certainly wasn't the best place for her. During her stay, Eileen would spend most of her time with me, or the enrichment coordinator who also worked at the care home. Eileen loved classical music and would join in on most of the music sessions I'd be conducting.

One fine afternoon after my group music session, I thought it a good idea to take Eileen for a spin in the car to the nearby garden centre. She immediately took to the idea of getting away from the care home for a while, and we chatted along quite happily and listened to some of her favourite music in the car.

When we arrived at the garden centre, Eileen immediately noticed a section at the centre that sold clothes, and in a highly excited manner proceeded to rush around picking up several items of clothing and accessories. It soon became clear to me that she wanted to buy the whole lot, which – including the three leather bags now in her arms – amounted to several hundred pounds!

I was getting very worried as to how this trip was going to end! As we walked towards the cashier, she shared some doubts about some of the items she'd accumulated; and to my relief, by the time we reached the cashier, she had thankfully reduced her shopping items down to the one handbag. There was a moment of panic when I thought that Eileen would not be able to remember the pin number for her card; but to her delight, she managed to retrieve this from her memory and walked away, smiling, having had – what was to her – a normal afternoon, resulting in a purchase of a lovely navy-blue leather handbag.

Having returned to the care home a little later, Eileen took great delight in transferring everything from her old handbag to her new leather acquisition, sorting out its contents while doing so. However, when I next came into work, Eileen was reunited with her old handbag, like an old friend. The new handbag was lying flat in the corner of her room having been discarded unceremoniously!

*****

Raymond has already been introduced to the reader in the chapter on 'Moon River' – the song to which he could remember all the words. As with Eileen, I knew that Raymond would also enjoy a trip in the car, but the combination of Parkinson's disease and Korsakoff Syndrome made it far trickier for me to persuade Raymond to come along.

It took many attempts and months of trying for the timing to be just right to take Raymond for the long-awaited drive. First, it had to be a sunny day, and it had to be a day when I was actually working at that home. It also had to be a period during the day when no group sessions were planned; and, above all, Raymond had to be in the right frame of mind to go for a ride, out of his self-imposed hibernation.

It was a beautiful late September afternoon. Most of the tourists who spent the summer months holidaying in the nearby town had finally returned home. A sudden calmness and stillness descended upon the beautiful area surrounding the care home where Raymond lived.

Nevertheless, it still felt like quite an event to finally take Raymond out for a drive in the car. The carers came to see him off, making sure he was comfortably seated, belted up and feeling warm enough. Photos were taken and there were plenty of smiles all around, especially from Raymond. Evidently it was going to be quite an adventure for him. Finally, we were off.

We drove into the nearby town, along its cobbled streets and narrow lanes towards the imposing historic castle that stood near the river's edge. Raymond insisted on having his window opened, 'to see it properly'. We drove past the marina so he could gaze at the beautiful yachts moored in neat rows next to one another, and the fishing boats in the bay with their gaggle of nets and lobster pots stacked higgledy-piggledy. Seagull cries could be heard punctuating the polyrhythmic clanging of the yacht's halyards.

Raymond drank in all the sights and sounds as if he was viewing them with new eyes. It must have felt to him that he was experiencing these sights for the very first time. He had lived most of his life in an area not far from the town we were visiting, and what we saw would almost certainly have been familiar to him from years gone by. In fact, he had previously told me that he'd frequented many of the pubs situated in this very town.

But that was all in a previous life. Now he was with me, gazing at the castle with awestruck eyes, stating, 'I've never seen this castle before, you know.' It was lovely being there with Raymond, sharing his excitement at seeing the castle as if for the first time. Yet the joy was also tinged with a sadness – the sadness of an unrecoverable past with its scrambled, scattered memories.

We took our time to take in all the sights before heading back to the care home. Raymond was warmly welcomed back into the fold, as if returning from a great voyage or epic adventure. He happily recounted what he'd seen to anyone who listened and was thoroughly enjoying all the attention he received from the carers. His parting words to me on that day was, 'When are we going again, nurse?'

*****

Driving along the river straits near the care home one afternoon, Mathew, who was also mentioned in the chapter called 'The Jazz Man and the Trumpet Man', was reminded of the time he used to go fishing.

He recounted the time when he used to use worms as bait. He would keep them in a little tin that contained wood shavings. 'I used to love fishing', he reflected. 'We'd catch trout'. He paused briefly for a moment before saying, 'I don't think we were supposed to, though!' To my delight, Mathew would recount our drive in the car for weeks and even months afterwards. He would say enthusiastically to visiting family and friends, 'There were mountains to the right of us and the straits to the left. The views were incredible!'

A few weeks later, at the end of a meeting with the owner of the care home, I recounted my little drive with Mathew to him, fearing perhaps that he might disapprove of my clandestine activities as a kind of 'unofficial-tour-guide-cum-musician-in-residence' for the residents. On the contrary, he thought it an excellent idea and even provided me with a pair of binoculars that I could take on such trips.

Mathew loved the fact that we had a pair of binoculars in the car. We would stop the car at various intervals so Mathew could take out the binoculars from its case. Holding them to his eyes and varying the focus, he would then take a closer look at the mountains, the fishermen in their boats on the straits, and the plethora of wildlife all around.

I could feel through Mathew that this felt to him like freedom – simply enjoying being in the moment, and then finally returning 'home' with the promise of tea and cake. More than anything, the car trips represented a kind of temporary return to normality for the residents who would come along. They often appeared far more at ease with themselves and their lives when they returned back to the care home.

19. The Dementia Ball Game

Putting on some fifties music to lightly play in the background, out came the unmistakable voices of Dean Martin, Frank Sinatra, Perry Como – the great crooners for the men in the lounge.

It was a grey afternoon, and so I'd suggested to the six gentleman residents that we'd have a game of Boccia. Boccia is similar to bowls but is often played by people with physical impairments; it is a sport that's played at the Paralympics. The balls are soft but quite heavy and have a faux leather exterior. There are six red balls and six blue balls and a smaller white ball which is used as a target.

I found it very interesting how residents with different types of dementia, and at different stages, played Boccia with various abilities that where unexpected and surprising to me.

Mathew, you met in Chapter 16, 'The Jazz Man and the Trumpet Man' – I could always have a decent conversation with him, we'd discuss the weather, he'd talk about his family who'd been visiting, he'd even ask me how I was and what I'd been up to since I last saw him. And of course, we'd have lengthy discussions about music. However, to my surprise, Mathew simply could not perceive the central white ball that needed to be aimed at with his own red ball. I noticed by looking at his eyes that he was focusing in a completely different direction to the white ball. Even when I stood up to stand near the white ball and point out this was the ball that was to be aimed at, Mathew continued to aim in a totally different direction. Considering that, to me, Mathew was the least affected by dementia, I found this quite unexpected.

However, Mathew was enjoying the game – what could I say…? Just, 'Well done! Fancy another round?'

Mathew had what is known as mixed dementia (see introduction). Symptoms would depend on the type of mixed dementia, for example a combination of Alzheimer's and Vascular dementia, where Alzheimer's would be predominant. The symptoms would therefore be very similar to Alzheimer's and these symptoms could well include impaired judgment, disorientation and difficulty performing spatial tasks – which could explain why Mathew was having difficulty aiming for the white target ball.

Another gentleman, called Alfie, whose conversation was quite limited, he seemed a little more confused and was confined to a special chair as walking had become very limited. However, Alfie completely understood the concept of the game and played very well. He even tried to help Mathew by telling him that he needed to aim for the white ball. He also enjoyed playing and was up for another game. Interestingly, Alfie had vascular dementia, and Parkinson's disease. Performing spatial tasks, therefore, might not be such a problem for Alfie.

Trevor, who had Alzheimer's, although he seemed to be able to focus on the central white ball, could not bring himself to release the ball from his hand. Though poised to do so, no amount of encouragement would make Trevor release the ball. The act of releasing the ball could simply not be triggered. Once again Alfie called out with encouraging comments from his chair, 'There you go, looking good, nearly there, just drop the ball!' Of course, this hampered somewhat with the flow of the game, and the other residents would get tired of waiting for their turn. In the end, they just took their turns sporadically resulting in balls rolling around the floor in all directions! In the end someone would call out at Trevor, 'Just throw the god-damn ball man!'

It seemed that, on the whole, residents who had vascular dementia performed better at Boccia than those with Alzheimer's or mixed dementia.

Each individual living with dementia is different, but I can't help wondering: do those individuals who are living with Alzheimer's have more difficulty in executing a move compared to those individuals living with vascular dementia? Even though some traits of both kinds of dementia are similar, for example, impaired judgment; playing a game such as Boccia highlights those individual traits in various types of dementia and at various stages of the disease.

One for the scientists!

20. A Different Me

As Benjamin twisted away to Chubby Checker's *Twist*, his daughter – thinking he was still in the lounge finishing his breakfast – stopped short by the music room door and did a double-take. She was looking on at her father with complete and utter incredulity. She couldn't believe that her quiet, reserved father was there, in front of her, dancing *The Twist*. And from the huge smile spread across his face, it looked as if he was actually enjoying the experience too!

I've often seen families looking very surprised at a photo I have taken during one of the 'Art in Response to Music' sessions, or of a loved one laughing while dancing to rock 'n' roll. They often come out with comments such as, 'He was never the slightest bit interested in painting!', or 'My mother dancing to rock 'n' roll? She hated it! In fact, she loved *opera*!'

Some residents who never used to paint would suddenly start enjoying painting, just as some residents who used to love rock 'n' roll might start listening to classical music, or vice versa. Strangely enough, while a PWD may initially refuse to take part because they feel that they are unable to do something that they used to be able to do before, it can also function as an emancipating and liberating force. Dementia may feel like it's a sign of the end, but it can also signal a new beginning. There are always new things to discover in life.

Dementia changes people. Different kinds of dementia can bring with it different symptoms. It can bring out what friends and relatives might consider as 'uncharacteristic' behaviour. A person may start using uncharacteristically aggressive language or may even start to speak a completely different language altogether (as mentioned earlier in Chapter 1, 'Hands on Music'). Physical aggressiveness is another common symptom of dementia. Loved ones can become characteristically inhibited – or the opposite – uncharacteristically uninhibited.

Symptoms of the most common forms of dementia such as Alzheimer's or vascular dementia causes people to become agitated and/or aggressive. In Korsakoff syndrome (or alcoholic dementia), symptoms can also include apathy (lack of interest, enthusiasm or concern), or at the other end of the spectrum, a person can become incredibly talkative, asking far too many questions.

I'm not saying that PWD's interests change completely with their illness: far from it. Most PWD will continue to love listening to their favourite music, will still love to dance. Conversely, they may continue to dislike, and therefore avoid, craftwork or baking cakes. But we must bear in mind that PWD's interests *can* change. We must not *assume* that their interests will remain unchanged or that their likes and dislikes will remain the same. If the PWD allows it, then music can be helpful because it is so varied and can be introduced in so many different ways.

We can listen to classical music (some will even 'conduct' along to a piece of classical music); we can dance to Elvis Presley; we can sing along to 'Danny Boy'; we can sing *with* Julie Andrews; we can exercise to Frank Sinatra; we can cry to Ella Fitzgerald; we can stand up and sing a Welsh hymn such as *Calon Lân* (Pure Heart) or 'Moon River' with evident passion and emotion, from the bottom of our hearts.

PWD must not be pushed into doing something they do not wish to do, just because *we* think they should, or that we think they might like it.

I've had relatives tell me that mothers or fathers who had never been volatile in the past had become increasingly physical and/or verbally aggressive since developing dementia. These unfortunate traits now became part of their character. However, it would sometimes work the other way. The daughter of a resident once told me that – before being diagnosed with dementia – she remembered her mother as being quite difficult, critical and strict with her. But since developing dementia, she had mellowed somewhat. She was warmer, gentler with her daughter, she did not seem so hard of heart. And her daughter, in turn, had truly come to value the time the two of them spent together, chatting and laughing and enjoying each other's company during the final chapter of her mother's life.

21. 'If they're not going to remember, why bother?'

On a bitterly cold evening a couple of weeks before Christmas we had a concert lined up, a charity event, and I was waiting anxiously for one of the performers – who was running late – to arrive. Residents had already congregated in the music room above the entrance to the care home, waiting for the concert to begin. Many family members were also present, in addition to carers, trustees and several other musicians who were taking part.

While I waited by the entrance to the care home, ready to let the performer in quickly from the cold, a relative was about to leave the care home after his weekly visit. Noting my increasing anxiety that the performer might not even turn up at all, he said offhandedly, 'Oh, I wouldn't worry. They're not going to remember a thing about it, anyway, are they?' And off he went into the night, chuckling away at his own remark.

I was quite surprised at his comment, especially since he had a relative in the home with dementia. I hope he will find time to read this book. Especially this chapter. And I hope he remembers what it says.

People with dementia may not necessarily remember what they sang during a session or even what they did; whether they danced or not, or what instruments – if any – were used. But if they enjoyed the session and it made them feel happy at the end, then certainly that feeling of happiness will be more likely to remain with them for most of the morning, afternoon or rest of the day.

We must remember when caring for PWD that it's the *moment* that counts for these people – what we do and how we feel in that moment. Yesterday and tomorrow means nothing to them. If we have a good session together for half an hour, or a whole hour, then we have achieved something together – a precious hour for them, perhaps; and if we're lucky, precious memories for us too.

However, I truly believe that some PWD *do* remember specific aspects of these music sessions, and also other day-to-day activities. For example, the movements to Perry Como's 'Catch a Falling Star', as mentioned in Chapter 10, or Mathew recalling the landmarks he saw during our drive in the car. Many residents will certainly recognise me as the person who conducts the music sessions. They'll often come out with comments such as, 'Oh, it's you! Are we having music today?'

Many years ago, I desperately wanted to prove that PWD could remember new things from one week to the next, and even that they could learn *new* things. But perhaps we should not focus too much on trying to examine aspects of 'cognitive function' during music or other sessions. As a person living with dementia herself, Christine Bryden's perspective attempts to consider the way PWD think. Often too much emphasis is placed on trying to help PWD remember. But perhaps we should be placing more emphasis on what is important to them, which is to live for the moment and to experience the enjoyment and emotion which can come from doing so. Maybe that's something we can all take on board in our lives.

Bryden's book is popular in this field because rarely do we come across a PWD write about their experiences of living with dementia. It therefore gives a valuable and rare insight into the lives of PWD. This is what Bryden has to say when discussing memory:

> *I usually enjoy each moment of our time together, so why is it so important that I remember it? Please keep visiting me, even if I might not remember that you came before, or even who you are. The emotion of your visit, the friendly feelings you give to me, are far more important. It is the emotion I connect to, not the cognitive awareness of the event.*

She goes on to state:

Why does it matter if I cannot remember, if I repeat myself, or forget what you told me. If I enjoy your visit, why must I remember it? Why must I remember who you are? Is this just to satisfy your own need for identity? Your visit is not a cognitive experience that I will store and recall. Let me live in the present. If I forget a pleasant memory, it does not mean it was not important to me.[35]

Of course, Bryden's comments do not reflect the view of all people living with dementia, but it certainly provides an insight into what is important to her and possibly many other PWD too.

I never feel negative about the fact that a music session will probably be forgotten very soon. You simply can't think in that way when working or spending time with PWD. And sometimes, as mentioned above, more often than you'd think, you'll find that PWD *do* remember things from one session to another, especially when those sessions involve music.

35   Christine Bryden, *Dancing with Dementia* (Jessica Kingsley Publishers, 2005), p. 110.

22. The White Lounge

There was a lounge in one nursing home where I worked where most of the residents, all female, were in the later stages of various forms of dementia. I called this lounge *The White Lounge*. Around twelve women would spend most of their time in this lounge. It was a noisy lounge, mainly because of the verbal noise. Some of the residents would shout aggressively. One or two would call or talk out loudly to themselves, due to the hallucinations they experienced. Others constantly repeated the same words over and over again. Dinner plates and cups were sometimes flung across the room; chairs and tables pushed and pulled noisily across the hard floor. The room seemed permanently on edge and often on the verge of descending into full-blown chaos.

At first, I found it difficult to conduct a music session in this environment. It was very hard to connect with the residents, either individually or collectively. The dementia had all but devoured their once lucid minds.

After a few disheartening attempts, where it was hard for me to hear myself above the unremitting din or concentrate on my music when having to swiftly dodge a flying teddy or a plastic cup, I decided one morning just to place myself in the centre of the lounge and play some gentle music on the harp. I interspersed this by occasionally singing some old Welsh love songs. The noise gradually subsided and the residents seemed calmer, more settled. After a little while, some comments were made by the residents. They were attempting to communicate their enjoyment. Those who were usually restless and verbal during this time of day would fall asleep peacefully.

The nurse came into the lounge to administer the medications as per usual. He saw that the residents seemed relaxed and settled. When his work was done in the lounge, he took a final look around him before declaring, 'You should come with me this evening when I'm administrating the meds. I often have real difficulty with some of the residents during this time. It's just so difficult coaxing them to take their meds with some residents getting quite aggressive.' Accompanying the nurse later that day, sure enough the medications seem to go down much better than usual whilst I played on the harp. Rather than 'a spoonfull of sugar helps the medicine go down', it was a case of a few relaxing melodies on the harp that helped the medicine go down that day!

One lady who resided in this lounge was called Phoebe. She did not have many visitors as most of her family now lived abroad. However, during one of the very few visits that she received, I was told that Phoebe used to be a beautiful singer and sang in a choir. Sadly, since her dementia had progressed, Phoebe hardly ever sang. But one curious feature of her dementia was that she sang when she was distressed.

She could be heard singing long, resonant, high notes as the carers raised her in the morning, washing her and getting her dressed. It would be the same when they would have to move her, as they'd need to use a hoist and wheelchair. It was as if she was singing in this way to cope with what she found difficult or unpleasant, such as personal care, or being moved.

Needless to say, Phoebe did not sing with me, but when I sang for her, I could sense a connection. I could also *see* a connection in her eyes. I also found sadness and tiredness in her eyes. Even though some of the residents would sleep for hours, many continued to look tired – tired of the confusion, tired of the loneliness, tired of simply being.

Whenever possible, I would ask one of the carers to bring one of the residents over to the music room where it would be quieter, but it was not always easy as most of the residents in *The White Lounge* needed to be hoisted. Also, even though it was noisy in the lounge, moving them could cause more distress in the end, and even despite my best intentions, there was always the possibility that they would not want to engage in any kind of musical event, be it a group or a one-to-one session.

The path where these people have travelled through their lives has cruelly crumbled away. Now there is no path. Missing all the coordinates and with no direction, they seem lost. Only confusion reigns. Occasionally there are stepping-stones, but these too crumble beneath them, into the abyss. Memories falter and fail as they flail around in their confusion, often desperate, lonely and unreachable.

23. Music to Die For

'Because I could not stop for Death –
He kindly stopped for me...'

(Emily Dickinson)

Work had been carried out by a Scottish drama company called Vanishing Point in conjunction with the Scottish Ensemble Orchestra, exploring the role of music at the end of one's life. Using the beautiful and compelling music of Estonian composer Arvo Pärt, they created a show that focused on one of his compositions, called *Tabula Rasa*.[36] Matthew Lenton, the director of Vanishing Point, had chosen *Tabula Rasa* because he'd read that many AIDS patients in New York hospices during the early 1990s had requested this music during their final hours. His assertion – based on direct accounts and some ground research – was not only that certain kinds of music could reach, touch and comfort people who were reaching the end of their lives, but that the person's own

---

36   Kate Molleson, "The last thing you'll ever hear: what is the world's best deathbed music?' *The Guardian*, 8 November 2017.

personal choice of music could also help enormously in such moments.

I was subsequently asked to contribute to a discussion on a radio program to talk about my own experiences of what music to play for people who are in their final hours. Why are certain kinds of music more appropriate than others? Should the music simply function as background accompaniment – a cosy, aural blanket of ambient comfort – or should it be more meaningful than this? Should it be there to touch the person personally – to form a bridge for the dying person on their journey from this world to the next, and guide them along it?

This is not an easy topic of conversation, mainly because I feel death is of course a very personal and private matter. And, as I reiterated on the radio program, I certainly did not want the music I might play to feel like an intrusion during those final hours. If a person is falling in and out of consciousness, how am I to know whether a certain piece of music – or any music at all – is welcome? I'm not even sure whether I'd want to hear some of my favourite music during my final hours.

However, there are a couple of contrasting examples and experiences I can draw upon when discussing this sensitive and difficult subject. If a close relative specifically requests that I play some gentle music on the harp during a loved one's final hours, then I will oblige. Usually, it will be for a person that I've have worked with closely in the care home over a period of months or years. I will know their music tastes, their likes and dislikes. The family might even request a specific song or piece of music.

The main aim of any music should be to comfort the dying, and if any relatives are also present, they too can draw comfort from it. With one particular lady, a nurse actually asked me to be by her side as the family were not going to make it in time. I can imagine that going through death can be a very lonely and bleak experience. It is, after all – ironically – the final, definitive act of one's life.

Another aspect to consider is that the music someone may want to hear during their final moments may also be the kind of music they would want others to hear at the funeral service, to remember them by. This might be a favourite hymn, folk-tune, song, or piece of classical music. But of course, one can never take this for granted. We can't just simply speculate. We could get it very wrong.

The lady to whom I was called by the nurse was semi-conscious, and I didn't know if she could hear me or not. I knew that she liked the old Welsh songs and so I played very gently on the little harp while she lay there in deep sleep. I did not sing to her; it didn't feel right to do so on this occasion. I had to trust my instincts in such situations.

When I returned to work the next day, the nurse informed me that the lady had passed away peacefully less than an hour after I left. I still don't know whether I had done the right thing or not by playing for her. If she could hear me, I hope I didn't intrude on her death.

Of course, it's a truism when people say that we have no control over our own death, unless we take it into our own hands. But I wonder if, during those final hours, one can actually retain some control? It often feels – in that strange liminal space between life and death – as if the person is waiting for something to happen before she or he lets go, before finally slipping away. Often it will seem as if they are waiting for loved ones to arrive. At other times they might want the opposite. They may be waiting for the family to leave – to be left alone – to shuffle off that mortal coil in peace.

A wife once came to ask me whether I'd come to sing for her husband. He didn't have long to live but he was awake, conscious and was sitting up in bed. We sang some songs that they had enjoyed singing over the course of their many years together. We smiled, we laughed, and we cried during the time I was with them. The whole atmosphere was relaxed and calm. Since the husband was awake, I could see from his response that this was a good, positive experience. They both sat listening while holding each other's hands.

When his wife left a little while after me, he slipped away quietly. His wife was distraught not to be with him when he passed away, as she had not expected him to die quite so soon. But in this instance, I'd like to think that perhaps he had waited for her to go, that he wanted her last memory of him to be one where he was awake and smiling, where he was able to say his goodbye to her.

Every person is different, and the process we go through when facing death will be different for each one of us. Just as music can soothe and comfort in life, it can also console in death, too. But not everyone will wish to appreciate music's healing powers. For some, music represents life, love and memories of happier days. When all those things have been lost, sometimes even the music vanishes too.

24. 'I Care for You'

Although this chapter does not discuss the role of music when working with PWD (apart from a few paragraphs at the end), I feel that I need to document my thoughts on carers who work in this field of care. I've come across a variety of carers over the years, some wonderful people, others not quite so. Four qualities are absolutely essential in making a good carer: empathy, respect, patience and kindness. These four characteristics are required in more-or-less equal measure. Take one of these elements out of the square and the balance is lost.

It's a sad but true fact that some people are totally unsuited to this role. Many are provided with adequate training skills via induction events, which are often conducted by companies who run the care homes. Empathy, respect, patience and kindness come mainly from within the person, however. I've often noticed a smile disappear from a carer's face once he or she has turned away from a resident. They are acting the part of the carer rather than actually living it. Residents with dementia can completely sense when a carer is being disingenuous.

The flip side of the coin is that I've often been full of admiration for many special carers, where the above qualities determine their character. Certainly, it's possible to teach a person empathy, respect, patience and kindness, but for some carers these four elements form the very fabric of their character and personality. Carers who work with those who have mid to late-stage dementia must deal with people who are often doubly incontinent, unable to feed themselves, who shout and who constantly repeat themselves. They require regular washing – a process often made more complex and difficult by the person's physical condition – and often have to placate seriously distressed residents who are fearful of, and resistant towards, any personal care.

Some carers can be very young, maybe just a year out of school. (The living wage is less to pay, so younger carers prove a cheaper alternative for employment.) I find it quite shocking what these young people must see and do with hardly any experience. Having said that, I've met young carers who demonstrate exceptional patience and are always respectful with residents. On the other hand, I have also met many young carers in tears, simply overwhelmed by the magnitude of it all, struggling with the demands of a difficult job and the prohibitively long hours involved. Even worse, I have witnessed complete indifference and lack of respect to a resident's circumstances from some carers. I no longer see empathy, respect and patience but apathy, disrespect, inattention and carelessness.

Good practice of care can be seen when, for example, carers prepare Raymond for his car trip with me, and the warm welcome he receives when we return. That kind of care makes Raymond feel special, and indeed loved.[37]

On several occasions I have entered a lounge to find the air conditioning racked up to the max as some of the carers are finding it too hot. Meanwhile the residents sit there shivering, stone cold and miserable in their chairs for hours. Another bugbear of mine is daytime TV heard blaring away in communal lounges. It will often feature a talk show, which usually consists of angry voices, arguing and shouting with fingers being pointed accusingly at each other. And all of this would go on for several hours at a volume too high, even, for the hard-of-hearing. To paraphrase Karl Marx, TV has now become the opium of the people. It's an easy fix for an impatient and negligent carer: simply switch on the TV, crank up the volume, and leave them to it.

What sort of ambiance does this create in a room? The first thing I feel the need to do when walking into a lounge is turn down the volume, then change the channel to a gardening or cookery show, maybe a show about re-decorating the home, otherwise I'd change the channel to a radio station that is playing some soothing classical music or light popular music. This is often greeted with distaste and disapproval from some carers but many of the residents will appreciate it.

How many times do some carers need reminding that this is the residence's home, not theirs? I can imagine that

---

37   See Chapter 12 'Moon River'.

some are not best pleased to see me fiddling with the TV remote in search of a more suitable TV program or radio station. Anyway, there is nothing as tiring and vacuous as a TV droning on in the background all day.

Care homes have to get out of the depressing fashion of switching on the TV first thing in the morning, assembling all the residents around it, and making it the focal point of their day. Of course, there is a time and place for TV, but absolutely not all day, every day. Conducting music sessions, art sessions or some kind of activity – even if it's just a board game or reading stories to residents – should be incorporated regularly into day-to-day care. Respect the residents and they will respect you.

It works both ways. Stick someone in front of the TV in an armchair in the corner of the room all day long and they're not going to be very responsive, chatty or in the best of moods come dinner time. Involve the same person in an array of different activities and most likely he or she will feel far more alert and receptive.

Some carers, while being efficient, can come across as being too authoritarian. Their attitude borders on behaviour that some might consider as 'bullying'. They will raise their voices and command things from others. They will become too forceful physically and verbally with residents during mealtimes: '…to drive them full-tilt upon their limitations…' as Oliver Sacks would say in his book *The Man Who Mistook his Wife for a Hat*. Residents are very sensitive to this kind of treatment, and I have noticed that those residents who can still walk will wonder away from the lounge in fear, away from the unsettling presence of a domineering carer.

When I revisit a care home after a few weeks elsewhere, I am often saddened to find out that one of the good carers no longer works there due to a combination of poor pay and exorbitantly long hours. Even worse is when I hear that a carer has left a home having voiced concerns about the safety and wellbeing of a resident on several occasions, and nothing has been done to address the problem. A conscientious and reliable carer may decide that he or she simply cannot continue to work under such circumstances.

The attitude of some owners and their management will often be that 'there are plenty more people out there who will take the work' and will release the disillusioned carer without even a second's thought. Letting go of reliable, experienced, and – above all – *caring* carers, with whom residents trust and know, is as short-sighted as it is retrogressive. Those at the top of the hierarchy and in a position of authority and control should listen to these people and take note of what they say. Rather than be swayed by financial concerns, they should try to see things from the carers point of view and try to learn from them. Above all, managers should do their utmost to encourage the best carers to stay on. Quality of care should always be the primary focus and concern of every care home. I have been very fortunate to receive unwavering support from my manager together with the owners of the dementia care centre where I'm mainly based as a Resident Musician.

They have always known and respected the value of music and enrichment in a dementia care setting.

Of course, in various homes, carers and nurses will often leave, having handed in long letters of resignation. There is a paper trail here … but how many people near the top of the pyramid are actually taking note of what is being said by them? Their concerns need to be properly addressed and discussed, especially if it will result in a better quality of life for the residents.

As I mentioned earlier in this book, residents may not remember what specifically occurred during a music or other session, but they will remember the feeling that comes with the session. In the same way, residents will remember how a carer makes them feel. These feelings can be good or bad, positive or negative. A carer can induce a feeling of comfort and reassurance, or, conversely, unease and uncertainty. Over time, many residents and carers will establish a bond that only close contact and good caring can provide. I've often seen a carer become very upset when a resident dies and will respectfully attend the funeral on behalf of the care home and in support of the resident's family and friends.

So, what should be the ideal situation regarding carers?

Finding the balance is very difficult. Most care homes and nursing homes conduct mandatory training and inductions which can give the impression that there's so much to cram in and remember. But the truth is that much of it is tangential and the really important issues – the crux of the care – gets sidelined. As I mentioned earlier, if a person decides that they want to be a carer then the most important things to remember are patience, empathy, respect. Finally, of course, and perhaps above all else, there is also kindness. Even in the face of residents whose dementia has made them very difficult to care for, one should always show kindness. If the above qualities are present, then many more good traits that are needed will fall into place.

Caring involves levels of selflessness rarely encountered in other walks of life. The well-known saying that 'patience is a virtue' is very fitting to the role of a carer as this is a skill required in abundance. It is so important to avoid becoming frustrated with residents. To be empathetic to the plight of these residents and their families will also make a good carer, as will constantly being kind and respectful – it is the very least the residents deserve.

Reassurance and words of kindness that might be forgotten in seconds will need to be reiterated repeatedly.

'I'm right here next to you, I'm not going away.'
'I'm here for you, I won't let you go.'
'You'll be okay, don't worry.'

These words and phrases can be easily forgotten in the challenging circumstances and conditions that a busy carer will find herself or himself. As I have said throughout this book: *always* seek the person *behind* the dementia. Never forget that each and every one of these people had a life. Many were incredibly important people who contributed much to the society in which they lived. Some were even carers or nurses themselves. Respect that life.

It may seem an obvious thing to say, but all residents in care homes and nursing homes once had a life. As evidenced by the colourful photos and images in their memory boxes, or in the stories they tell, many experienced very colourful and eventful lives. I've met people who used to be teachers or university lecturers. Some were in the armed forces during the war. Others were politicians, athletes, ministers, chefs, bankers, doctors or nurses, busy housewives. And many, many were nurses.

In contrast, their present life no longer has a clear direction. Their existence can no longer be called a 'life' in the true sense of the word. All that they can do now is to take each day as it comes, and our role is to make each day as full and complete for them as we can. As for the future? The future has cruelly been taken away from them by their dementia. They can no longer look into the future with hopes and dreams.[38]

During my music sessions, I dissuade carers from removing residents from the sessions if they become upset during certain songs as some songs evoke feelings

---

38 I would like to think that they can still experience lucid dreams, where they escape, free from the confusion and angst of their living days. Where they no longer feel afraid or uncertain. I hope they can still experience happiness in their dreams.

of longing. It is not a 'bad' thing to feel sad. There are also many songs that bring joy and fun. However, if a resident becomes particularly distressed or upset during a session, then it may be beneficial for them not to stay, but only before being reassured first of all. It may well be that some residents will not be having such a good day and might benefit from attending a session another day.

And finally, we need to challenge and change elitist perceptions about music that still exists when it comes to music provision at care homes. This may come as a shock to some, but you do not have to be a musician or a music therapist to use music in the care home. It's high time these deeply engrained highbrow perceptions about music held by the so-called guardians of 'musical taste' are dispelled once and for all.

The focal point should always be the resident and not the performer. Indeed, I'd go further and argue the quality of performance shouldn't always be the most important element either. Being able to connect and communicate is just as important, if not more so.

To give an example, a few years ago I was invited into a care home in south Wales where a professional harpist and soprano had come to perform for the residents, all living with some form of dementia. The performance was of excellent quality. However, when a gentleman resident got up to dance to the music, the soprano tried to accommodate this unexpected turn of events. When the song came to an end, she kindly informed the resident that he could return to his seat, but she couldn't comprehend why he continued to stand there. She failed to see that the resident could not remember where he'd been siting and needed assistance to guide him back to where he was seated. These are the little things that need consideration, and the little things are important.

I once read with interest a few years ago about an 'innovative' collaborative project between a high-profile University and several local dementia care homes. The project had received generous funding support from several institutions and research councils. It also received a lot of media attention and exposure at a time when dementia headlines were appearing regularly in newspapers and on the news.

When I read further about the project, I saw that it involved a professional singer visiting each care home in turn, interacting with residents, recording the sessions themselves and collecting quantitative and qualitative data. It all sounded very exciting until I discovered that the whole focus of the project was not on the effect of the music on the residents themselves but rather on the impact that those sessions were having on the performer!

To me, turning the focus on the performer – however important he or she may have been in this two way process – seemed a completely back-to-front way of doing things. I suspect that it was probably done this way in order to avoid obtaining all the necessary permissions, ethics and consent forms required from the resident's families. Yet that reason alone hardly justified the money spent or did little to validate the project's main aims and objectives.

The organisers of such projects need to think ahead and to see what provision there can be when a project ends. To educate care homes, to show how singing sessions can be adapted and to continue. There's not much point making a big splash, reflect in the glory of a successful project, then walk away, leaving the care homes with an empty void. Help the carers by showing them how the void can be filled, re-visit occasionally – all a crucial part of any such project.

The focus should be on the residents themselves. By conducting a little bit of research through asking each one and their family and friends what music they mostly enjoy, it's possible to gather together a simple repertoire and then enjoy a little singsong. Song sheets can be printed out if needed. Accompaniment is not absolutely necessary. You just need a carer with an extra smattering of self-confidence, who is just happy to sing and focus on the enjoyment rather than on the standard of singing. At the end of the day, the social benefits of collective singing far outweigh anything else. It's not always necessary to enlist the services of a famous opera singer to enrich the lives of PWD.

Also, try to keep these little informal singing sessions as a regular occurrence. Just twenty minutes or so every few days is much better than longer sessions that are conducted weeks apart with nothing much in-between.

Add a little light movement to the sessions if you think it will work. You'll find that many residents will remember from one session to the next and will start looking forward to them. It will become a welcome part of their routine. Even though, at times, it can get slightly tiring for me to sing the same songs week in, week out to the residents living with dementia, it must be remembered that familiar songs are a comfort. They often remember the melody and the words, it's one of the few things they can retain, therefore it's important to maintain the old favourites.

Large or small, old or new, there is no reason why music cannot be conducted in all dementia care homes across the country on a regular basis. Each session will enrich residents' lives no end. It may not cure the residents' dementia, but it will certainly make their lives far more rewarding and fulfilling as a result.

25. Singing and Smiling through Lockdown[39]

When the pandemic came, all the freelance music sessions I was doing came to an abrupt end, apart from conducting online zoom sessions, which were far from ideal. I was fully expecting a phone call or email from where I worked as a Resident Musician saying that I couldn't work for the time being at the home considering the circumstances. But it turned out instead that my job had become more important than ever.

Seeing so many of my peers experience their work drying up, I was acutely aware of how lucky I was to continue working. Part of my job as Musician in Residence was to organise outside entertainment to come to the home, and I had built up many great contacts who visited regularly: choirs, the local arts centre, a dance company, local primary and nursery schools, to name just a few. The home had a spacious music room, and we were used

---

39 This chapter is based on an article I wrote for *The Journal of Dementia Care,* September/October 2021 Vol. 29, No. 5.

to welcoming all the choirs until the music room was bursting with music!

I had to pull the plug on all of this straight away. Plus, we could not bring the residents together into the music room as one big crowd. The care home had been divided into 12 lounges with approximately nine residents in each lounge. Movement between lounges had to be restricted in case of a possible Covid-19 infection.

Thinking afresh, I had to think of an idea of how to deliver live music safely to the residents. By liaising with a few local schools, I managed to acquire four unused school pianos and placed them at strategic locations in the home; the grand piano in the music room that used to accompany the choirs had to be idle for now.

I also used my Celtic harp during the mini-music sessions. Strict rules had to be adhered to, so a mask, visor, and a bucket of anti-bacterial wipes became my daily tools as well as changing my clothes on arriving and leaving the care home. These mini-music sessions became an opportunity for me to get to know more of the residents and their taste in music and my aim was to make sure each lounge could experience some live music every week.

The news frequently focused on the frustration and anxiety felt by families in not being able to visit their loved ones for periods that felt cruelly long. They found talking over the phone, or even on FaceTime, hard to do when residents were sometimes unable to recognise their voices or even their faces on screen.

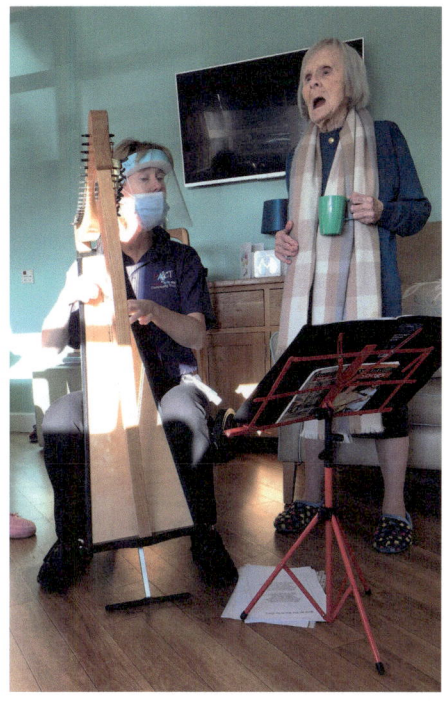

Yet the ability to sing remains with most people with dementia, and so we found a way of connecting. It was pure pleasure to hear tears of joy from one daughter as her father sang the popular Welsh hymn *'Calon Lân'* down the phone while I accompanied him on piano. Another man sang *'Bugeilio'r Gwenith Gwyn'* ('Watching the White Wheat') to the harp's accompaniment while his son watched and listened through FaceTime. This was a special way of connecting – often the only way – and families found it invaluable.

I got proposals from outside the home to participate in online concerts, but this kind of digital engagement was often a challenge too far for our residents. Instead, our home continued to sing and smile throughout the pandemic and, slowly, we came out of this distressing and frustrating time. The staff at the home worked as one big family, and fortunately there were only a few Covid cases, something I put down to a combination of sticking to the rules and a good dose of luck!

26. Epilogue

What would I say to myself if I knew that, someday, I would be facing a diagnosis of some form of dementia? Perhaps it's an impossible question to answer, but there are certainly some important things that spring to mind. To let go of any worries would definitely be one nugget of advice, although this is much easier said than done. Worrying can eat away at any hope of living well with dementia. Those who manage to set their worries aside are naturally more at peace with themselves and those around them. Live in the moment is another piece of advice I'd give myself, which is all you can do under the circumstances. Without the constant worries looping through one's mind, this can be easier.

In this book I have tried to show that musical ability is one of the very few things that remains preserved in people living with dementia. It is therefore vitally important to try to incorporate music into the daily lives of the ones we care for, using music to reopen avenues of communication and connection.

Music sessions can contribute to a better quality of life amongst PWD by stimulating present abilities, including neurological processes. It is extremely important that such sessions should continue and develop, and every effort made to make such activities an integral part of the weekly lives of people with dementia and for those who care for them.

Through working with PWD, I have found that their treasured memories become part of my memories. And, like them, some memories stand out as being clearer and more vivid than others. Likewise, some of these memories will probably never leave me. They have left their mark and are a reminder of how fortunate I have been to be able to share with them in the special memories that are often retrieved through a song.

But can our memories be trusted? Apparently not. Recent research claims that you can't always trust your memory. For example, two childhood friends in the same place at the same time may remember certain events, circumstances and details very differently many years down the line. One friend may remember that the boy on the school trip who fell and broke his arm had ginger hair and freckles. The other friend may recollect clearly that the same boy in fact had broken his thumb and had blond hair. We may think that we can remember things clearly, but it might surprise us to find out that they are not as accurate as we may think. However way we remember, does it really matter whether these memories are entirely accurate memories or not?

Whether they are accurate or not, memories can still provide a comfort to us. Many of us choose to forget some things, unpleasant or painful memories; some of us will experience dissociative amnesia[40] where painful memories from a long time ago stay buried until a disease such as Alzheimer's cruelly uncovers and exposes them, adding further to a person's confusion and grief.

I think of treasured memories as not only carried by, and in, the mind, but also carried in the heart. Memories are this special synthesis of mind and body, head and heart. In the words of Adriana Cavarero: 'Memory resides in the aria of the heartstrings as well'. We think of memories as consisting of visual or aural imprints of things that took place in the past. But memories also carry with them feelings and emotions. Memories can stir the emotions. It is vitally important that PWD, with help, continue to tap into their memory banks – an archaeology of memories. Music is often the key that allows us to unlock this vast reservoir, thereby bringing back the past into their lives in order to enrich the present.

---

40 A disorder that causes a person to be unable to remember important personal information, usually due to a traumatic or stressful event.

Acknowledgements

I wish to express my gratitude to Gill and Mario Kreft at Pendine Park Care for their passion in developing the arts in the care sector, and for their vision of employing a Resident Musician at Bryn Seiont Newydd care home. I have been supported throughout my time at Bryn Seiont Newydd by Sandra Evans, Anne Quinn Jones, and all the staff who have worked there, especially Emyr, Elliw, Audrey and Angela.

Several other care homes have played an important part in my work over many years, too many to name! My thanks also goes out to the following people for their support and positive influence: Sarah Edwards, Edwin Humphreys, my daughter Hawys for realising the book design idea, my husband Pwyll ap Siôn for his input; to the schools, their pupils and teachers, who have enriched many residents' lives; to the many choirs and musicians who have performed at various care homes; to dance company Dawns i Bawb, theatre company Theatr Frân Wen, the William Mathias Music Centre (diolch Meinir!); and above all, to the families and friends of the residents who have given their support, trust and consent. Diolch o galon i chi gyd!

About the Author

Originally from the Llŷn Peninsula, North Wales, Nia Davies Williams graduated in Music at Bangor University. She followed this with a masters' degree that focused on the relationship between music and dementia.

For three years, she coordinated 'Singing for the Brain' groups organised by the Alzheimer's Society in North Wales. Since then, she has delivered a pilot project using the arts to tackle loneliness among older people in rural areas throughout Gwynedd through a locally-based music centre[41] funded by the local council's community arts unit. Due to the initial success of the project, further sessions were funded and other areas of loneliness targeted in this region of Wales.

In addition to numerous freelance work in care homes around north and west Wales, working mainly with people who have dementia, Nia was made Resident Musician at Bryn Seiont Newydd Dementia Care Centre in 2015, which is part of the Pendine Park Care organisation in Wrexham, North Wales.

---

41   The William Mathias Music Centre is based in Galeri Arts Centre, Caernarfon, North Wales.

She has given presentations on music and dementia in several conferences in the UK and in the USA, publishing two articles in the multi-disciplinary Welsh-language online journal *Gwerddon*, both of which assess the effects of music on people who have dementia. She has also written articles on her work for *The Journal of Dementia Care.* In 2017 she was awarded the prestigious Sir Bryn Terfel Foundation Wales Care Award for Promoting the Arts in Social Care.